ROCK ON
POWER, SEX & MONEY AFTER SIXTY

STELLA FOSSE

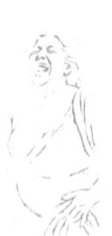

Copyright © 2025 by Stella Fosse

All rights reserved.

No part of this book may be reproduced in any form or by any electronic or mechanical means, including information storage and retrieval systems, without prior written permission from the author, except for the use of brief quotations in a book review.

ISBN 978-1-950227-13-6

Cover by Diana Rosinus (www.dianarosinus.com)

Versions of some material in this book previously appeared in these publications:

CrunchyTales Magazine

Liberté

Girl on the Net

This Age Thing

Starts at Sixty

Creative Crones Substack

The Stella Fosse Blog

Published by:

Baubo Books

400 Glen Creek Rd. NW #5120

Salem OR 97304-3060, USA

www.stellafosse.com

ALSO BY STELLA FOSSE

Write & Sell a Well-Seasoned Romance

Vampires of a Certain Age

Brilliant Charming Bastard

The Erotic Pandemic Collection

Aphrodite's Pen:
The Power of Writing Erotica After Midlife

To Graham
Who makes all things possible

CONTENTS

Introduction: Ten Things to Know in Your Sixties   xi

PART ONE
POWER

1. Gendered Ageism   3
2. Embracing Freedom   7
3. Becoming Age-Positive   15
4. By Any Other Name   19
5. Power Profile   23

PART TWO
CREATIVITY

6. Why a Debut Novel at Age 68?   29
7. The Crone Renaissance   33
8. Blood and Ink   39
9. The Unfettered Bliss of Trying Something New   49
10. Creativity Profile   53

PART THREE
SEXUALITY

11. Passion Abides   57
12. Sexual Agency after Sixty   61
13. The Nitty Gritty   65
14. Top Ten Reasons Why Women Over Sixty Should Write Erotica   73
15. Sexuality Profile   77

PART FOUR
HEALTHCARE

16. Manage Your Healthcare   81
17. Drugs after Sixty - Not the Fun Kind   89
18. Fear Sells   97
19. The Lowdown on Hormone Therapy   103
20. Healthcare Profile   111

PART FIVE
BODY

21. From Body Neutrality to Body Love	115
22. Now You See Her, Now You Don't	119
23. If Thy Uterus Offend Thee	123
24. To Be Fit, Old, and Fat	127
25. Body Profile	135

PART SIX
BEAUTY

26. Let She Who Grows Her Chin Hairs Cast the First Stone	139
27. Toward A New Definition of Beauty	143
28. The Legs are the Last to Go	147
29. The Tale of the Peacock	151
30. Beauty Profile	153

PART SEVEN
MONEY

31. Work Sucks for Women Too	159
32. Financial Strategies after Sixty	163
33. Medicare for Some	175
34. The New Improved Pink Tax	181
35. Money Profile	185

PART EIGHT
PURPOSE

36. The Grandmother Hypothesis	189
37. Including Ourselves in the Circle of Care	193
38. OK Big Oil	197
39. The Power of Late Bloomers	201
40. Purpose Profile	205

PART NINE
CULTURE

41. Once Upon Our Time	209
42. Oldfluencers	213
43. The Vibrant Pen	219
44. See It Then Be It	225
45. Culture Profile	231

PART TEN
SPIRIT

46. Retirement Till the End	235
47. A Life in Review	241
48. Speaking bawdy of the dead	245
49. My Next Life Bucket List	249
50. Spirit Profile	253
Epilogue	255
Questions to Think, Write, and Talk About	257
For Further Reading	263
Acknowledgments	267
About the Author	269

INTRODUCTION: TEN THINGS TO KNOW IN YOUR SIXTIES

Aging happens, because we cannot stop it, and it is not what we feared.

—Victoria Smith, *Hags*

On the morning of my sixtieth birthday, I walked with my firstborn to a breakfast cafe in Berkeley, CA. "It's funny," I said. "I don't feel old. I feel great."

My son looked down at me and smiled. "I'll tell you something that will make you feel old: You're going to be a grandma."

My granddaughter's pending arrival didn't make me feel decrepit or demented or any of the other nasty messages we get about aging. Nothing could have. The discrepancy between those stereotypes and the vivid life I led was too stark. I swam four times a week, I had lovers and a successful career, most of my kids were grown, and my health was great. I had switched teams from Princess to Crone; why

INTRODUCTION: TEN THINGS TO KNOW IN YOUR SIXTIES

was my life so different than the frail and forgetful olders in the media?

The party that night was raucous and fun (including my daughters' ill-advised attempt to persuade me to try weed). But no one handed me a roadmap to navigate the realities of a decade that would be transformative, in very different ways than society predicts.

Ten years later I turned seventy: another raucous party. This time I danced to loud rock-and-roll with four grandchildren. The decade of my sixties had been terrific. I'd graduated from my corporate career to live my dream of writing and publishing books. I'd met my wonderful partner and we had settled in a lovely home in a new state. All four of my children were launched and doing well. As I look back on my confusion about turning sixty and what I learned over the next ten years these ideas would have been a great introduction to that secretly wonderful decade:

1. **Do not let the future be the enemy of the present.** Every living creature, no matter their age, owes the universe a death. Yours may be collected tomorrow or decades from now. Worrying doesn't change it, and it's not your job to carry other people's fears. Your remaining years may be longer than the entire average lifespan of a human in the Middle Ages.

2. Remember the words of the immortal Maggie Kuhn, crone foremother and founder of the Gray Panthers: *Learning and sex until rigor mortis.* Both of these—curiosity and sexuality—are foundational. We grow and change throughout life; after sixty is our chance to explore new skills and ideas. What would you like to learn that you've never had time to study? And sexuality is our birthright. It is not a gift or burden imposed by the male gaze, but rather is innate to each of us. How we use our libidinal energy is our choice. We may have sex with another, or have solo sex, or channel that energy into play and creativity, or all three.

INTRODUCTION: TEN THINGS TO KNOW IN YOUR SIXTIES

3. **Creativity is now your superpower.** Reclaiming play is one of the great joys of life after sixty. All the bliss you've experienced, all the sorrow, every unexpected turn of fate—it's all material for your art. You are at peak creative power. And each vivid story you write, each vibrant painting you make, puts the lie to gendered ageism.

4. **We define our own aesthetic.** There is no need to buy into conventional ideas of beauty or fashion. We can make up our own. You might choose to be invisible on a Tuesday, and by Wednesday you're decked out like Iris Apfel. And how you, or any other woman, presents herself deserves all our respect.

5. **This is your chance to pay it forward**. Those of us who are privileged with freedom from work can help redress the inequities that keep other older women down. Women who provided unpaid labor to their families for decades and were underpaid when they worked outside the home deserve to live with dignity in their later years. We can advocate for public policies that provide older women with security in keeping with all they have contributed. We can volunteer and provide financial support.

6. **The paradox of aging is that there are losses and gains**. Society focuses on the losses; we can focus on the gains: the perspectives our long lives provide, the shedding of early conditioning and shame, and the reclamation of our time. As Leonard Cohen said, "Ring the bells that still can ring."

7. **The U-Shaped Happiness Curve is real**. Yes, we really are happier after sixty. That's because in our sixties we regain our freedom. So follow your bliss: Do the things you were put on this planet to do. It's about time you put yourself first. If you are able to retire, embrace it as soon as you can. And before you do, take time to consider what this epic part of life will be about.

INTRODUCTION: TEN THINGS TO KNOW IN YOUR SIXTIES

8. **The challenges you'll encounter have workarounds.** Yes, we might have less energy. Yes, there is medical gendered ageism. Yes, there's that old bugaboo, invisibility. There are ways to manage all of that, leaving us time for the really important work of whatever the hell we want.

9. **Every princess grows into a (supposedly wicked) witch whose real name is CronePower.** Think Maleficent but with a sense of humor and a gym membership. This is a lesson we can pass on to our daughters when it's their turn: Young and beautiful is all well and good; old and powerful is better.

10. **We are more powerful together.** Immerse yourself in Crone Culture: Read books by older women. Listen to podcasts that feature older women. If you're strapped, consider Golden Girls housing. Find your posse. Let's pay attention to each other, and invite the Apprentice Crones to join us.

Those are some highlights of what I wish someone had told my newly minted sixty-year-old self. And that's just the start. More to come—much more—in the chapters ahead.

May this book inspire your coming adventures.

Cheers,

Stella

INTRODUCTION: TEN THINGS TO KNOW IN YOUR SIXTIES

Where to Find Things in This Book

Each of the ten sections (Power, Creativity, etc.) includes four chapters that explore the topic, plus a profile of a woman who has catalyzed change in that arena.

At the end of the book is a list of *Questions to Think, Write and Talk About* for each topic. Grab a notebook and write your thoughts, or discuss with your book group, or both. Contact for my publicist is there too, in case you'd like to invite me to talk with your book group. I hope you will!

Finally, there's a list of references *For Further Reading*, in case you'd like to explore each topic in more depth.

PART ONE
POWER

To be realistic about aging means letting go of the ageist stereotypes we have encountered since childhood. We free ourselves to set our own priorities and enjoy all that the years ahead have to offer: our connections with others, our creativity, and much more.

The essays in this section explore the challenges and rewards of embracing our power in this phase of life.

CHAPTER 1
GENDERED AGEISM

Picture a graph with time across the bottom axis, from Birth to Death. The vertical axis shows happiness, with Unhappy at the bottom and Very Happy at the top. You might not expect what the research shows: A U-shaped happiness curve that looks like a smile, with happiness highest in childhood and later in life. Happiest of all is the decade of our sixties, despite the nonsense we've been told.

We have dealt with sexism from early childhood, when we watched beautiful passive Disney princesses being rescued from older women villains. Early in our work lives we were channeled into lower paid careers befitting the traits we were presumed to have (and to lack) as females.

Then to top it all off, along came ageism. Geena Davis, star of *Thelma and Louise* and many other films, thought her career was too big to be affected by ageism. Then on her fortieth birthday the phone calls stopped. Davis knew that male actors her age were getting roles well into their fifties. She believes that representation of olders in

Hollywood both reflects and reinforces stereotypes. She founded the Geena Davis Institute to study representation in the media, including representation of people of color, characters with disabilities, LGBTQ+ characters, and women. In 2021 the Institute published a study showing that women characters over fifty are seldom seen onscreen and are even rarer in lead and romantic roles.

The ageism we face has real impacts. Lifespans are longer in societies where older people are revered. And for women it's a double whammy: Ageism and sexism compound each other in unexpected ways. For older women of color and for older women with disabilities, those differences from the dominant paradigm complicate the picture even more.

Given the incessant stereotypes we have been exposed to, it's no surprise that gendered ageism exists within us as well as outside us. Both external and internal bias affect us in negative ways. In one example of external bias, studies show that older women have more difficulty accessing adequate healthcare than older men or younger women. But our health is also affected by our own views. Studies show that women with positive attitudes about aging live longer and healthier lives.

Our attitude is something that we have the power to control. We can decide what we want from life after sixty. The choices we make about everything from how much we exercise to what books we read change our lived experience. Improving our view of ourselves improves our health, happiness and well-being.

As for structural ageism, each of us individually may not control society's attitudes. But there are more older women in the United

States right now than there have ever been. As we each take charge of our own destiny, we help turn the tide for society at large. The essays in this book are about changing our own stories, and ultimately changing the future for more and more women who follow in our footsteps. Claiming our stories means claiming our freedom.

CHAPTER 2
EMBRACING FREEDOM

We spend much of our adult lives racing around like headless chickens. Sadly, the entry of most American women into full-time employment, which happened in our lifetimes, did not mean that spouses took on half the unpaid toil of keeping house and raising children. Plus the greater supply of labor in the workforce led to lower real wages across the board. Soon two incomes were needed to support a family in any sort of comfort. Women became trapped in that dual role of worker and homemaker, the Faustian bargain that second wave feminists made to attain economic freedom for women in the United States. To this day, many heterosexual couples with children rely on the woman to keep it all going once her paid workday is through.

For many of us the whole catastrophe resolves in our sixties. When the children grow up and our careers wind down, the occasional load of laundry is all that remains of the trifecta of kids, work, and home that we carried for so long.

You might expect women to greet that liberation with open arms. Many of us react like a seventh grader on the first day of summer break. The world opens up: Wilderness trails await our wandering feet. New recipes tempt us. Political campaigns welcome our volunteer energy. We fill galleries with our paintings and beguile readers with our books. Every dream we postponed during those too-busy years is suddenly right in front of us.

Yet for many women the prospect of an empty nest and life without a career is frightening. When I encourage women to reconnect with their dreams, I often hear some version of "I've focused on job and family for so long that I don't know what my dreams are."

Due to pay discrimination and the time many of us spend away from the workforce caring for young children, the average American woman approaches retirement with less savings than the average man—and must stretch those dollars over a longer lifespan. But existential dread can be just as real as money worries. Here are some of the questions women voice about life after sixty:

- **Fear of loss of status:** *I'm already less visible as an older woman. Who am I without my career? Who am I with an empty nest? What will I say when people ask, "What do you do?"*
- **Fear of loss of social connections:** *Most of my daily conversation is with coworkers. And I know how it goes when someone leaves a job: Folks plan to keep in touch but over time those connections fade.*
- **Fear of loss of purpose:** *I've been taking care of everyone, at home, at work, for decades. What is the point of my life when that stops?*

How to counteract these fundamental fears and enjoy a powerful next phase of life? First, let's recognize that these concerns are normal. For many of us, life after sixty means a big loss of structure, of all that is familiar, and it's only natural to feel unmoored. These days "retirement" means different things to different people. Some of us keep working, full-time, part-time, or as consultants. Some switch to a more fulfilling line of work or become writers or artists. But for most of us life after sixty includes a big shift in how we spend our days.

Lay the Foundations Before You Retire

Stepping back from full-time employment can be a process, not an event that happens on one particular day. We can lay the foundations for enduring purpose and connection months or years before that last day of work. If you are at that stage, try some or all of these steps.

Notice What Brings You Joy:

- Look back at your calendar for the past year. What did you do that you particularly enjoyed? What events did you miss that you wish you'd had time for?
- Look at a catalog for your local branch of the Osher Lifelong Learning Institute (or other local learning resources). What courses appeal to you, as something new you'd like to learn?

Make Peace with Your Inner Critic:

- Whether we love or hate our line of work, we're probably pretty comfortable doing it by now. Part of the fear of

retirement is worry about trying new things. The best advice I've seen: "Be ready to suck at something new."
- Before you retire, try at least one creative project you've never done before but where you're unlikely to judge yourself (collaging, anyone?).

Commit (or Recommit) to a Movement Practice:

- What types of movement bring you joy? Could be hiking, swimming, or just dancing in your living room.
- Make time for movement a couple times a week while you're still working, and plan to increase that once you retire.
- As our schedules open up we can care for ourselves with the same nurturing spirit we've offered to others. Besides movement, what other forms of self-care might bring you joy? Eating more vegetables? Keeping up with dental work? Playing piano?

Explore Ways to Redefine Purpose

There are many choices to build purpose in our lives that have nothing to do with the jobs we leave when we retire.

- Your purpose after retirement may involve creative skills you have now or want to develop. What forms of creativity appeal to you? Interest is foundational; skills can be learned.
- Brainstorm ways to use your interests and skills in the service of others. Could be volunteer work, or a part-time job that appeals to you. Your form of service may involve

writing or teaching; you may even decide to start a business that uses your talents.
- Explore ways to give back. Take a personal inventory of your interests, and of the skills you developed during your career. What do you bring to the table?

Build Social Networks Outside of Work

- As you prepare to retire, reconnect with friends you've been too busy to see. If they are about the same age, they may also be ready to rebuild networks.
- Consider activities that bring you into contact with people with shared interests. Could be a meditation group, an artists' collective, or a water aerobics class. What grabs you?

Once You Leave Full-time Employment

Suddenly the big day is here, often followed by catching up on a backlog of necessary rest. Then it's time for reinvention.

Push Back on Internal Ageism

As we start our retirement, the ageist messages we've internalized all our lives may come back to bite us. "Over the hill," "Senior moment," "OK Boomer," you know the drill. Don't feed those messages. Instead, embrace the freedoms you enjoy. What other people think of you is now irrelevant. Think of yourself as sexy and unleashed.

Define Your Post-Retirement Identity

Consider what you are learning about yourself. Who are you now? An artist? A teacher? A writer? (You get to claim what you aspire to be. If you've written a grocery list, you're a writer.)

- Brainstorm new answers to the question, "What do you do?" Practice an answer that reflects your new goals.
- Start a LinkedIn page (or revise your existing page) to show your new endeavors. Connect with people in similar roles and support them.
- Order post-retirement business cards that express your new direction.

Structure Your Time

Throughout those Second Shift years filled with career, family and household, our calendars booked themselves. One of the best and yet most daunting things about post-career life is that we control our own schedule. So take a deep breath and start with the big stuff.

I'm a fan of the Franklin-Covey Big Rocks method. Imagine you have four glass containers. One is empty; that represents the week you're about to plan. One contains big rocks (representing your top priorities), one contains medium rocks (your medium priorities), and one contains gravel (the nitty-gritty of daily life). If you fill the empty container with gravel, there is no room for the big rocks. But if you start with the big rocks, then add the medium rocks and finally the gravel, you'll end up focused on your top priorities and filling in with the lower ones.

Think about what you have learned through self-inventory and brainstorming, and choose three Big Rocks: your top priorities. At first your top goal might be recuperating from a lifetime of work, but your Big Rocks will change as your energy returns.

At the start of each week, map out roughly what you will do each day, including:

- **Big Rocks:** What will you do this week in line with the purposes you've defined for your retirement?
- **Self-Care:** Some form of movement each day, with more vigorous movement 3-4 times a week. What other self-care will you do this week? (Hint: Relaxation counts as self-care.)
- **Social Connections:** How will you interact with others each day? Could be a phone call about a shared volunteer effort, or perhaps you'll attend a class.

At the beginning of each day, get granular about the tasks and activities you'll set, in line with your goals, self-care, and connections with others.

In our work life, many of us wished for shorter hours and more time off. So it may seem paradoxical that many women dread the approach of retirement. Yet it's only natural when the road ahead is undefined. To embrace the freedom of our post-career life requires us to re-learn who we are and what we most want. Freedom means using the power to plan our time to meet the goals we set for ourselves.

It's a journey well worth taking: the journey to freedom and power in our sixties and beyond. And giving ourselves positive messages along the way is essential.

CHAPTER 3
BECOMING AGE-POSITIVE

Ever since childhood, we in the United States have been subjected to negative messages about olders. Even though we ourselves are now older and wiser, it is no surprise when we still harbor these thoughts. Remember "Never trust anyone over thirty?" Now that's us. Remember Martha Mitchell, the "crazy old lady" of the Watergate era? It turns out Martha was trying to blow the whistle on Richard Nixon and was drugged, kidnapped, and vilified for her trouble. Even now, when older women gather on social media to laugh at self-putdowns, internal ageism is at work.

Internal ageist and sexist bias can stop us from living our lives to the fullest. Dr. Becca Levy at the Yale School of Public Health ran a study in which one group of older adults was given negative prompts about aging and the other group was given positive prompts. Those who had received positive prompts walked better, were more sociable, and were more curious. And the longer the study went on, the more those positive messages were repeated, the more of a difference those messages made. It makes sense that repetition mattered, because the positive messages had to counter a lifetime of negatives.

We can do this work for ourselves. We can intentionally counteract the negative messages about aging that we have absorbed throughout our lives. Pay attention to the words you use and the ways that you explain your actions to yourself and others. If a woman has occasionally misplaced her keys since her twenties, losing them today is not suddenly evidence of dementia. If you start to tell yourself something negative based on age, turn it around. Instead of tearing yourself down, build yourself up.

It also matters what we tell ourselves about our abilities. Psychological studies over the past thirty years show that what we say to ourselves informs and predicts our behavior. Self-talk is an important way human beings regulate our emotions. When we give ourselves positive messages about an ability, we are more likely to perform well and to feel positively about how we perform, whether we outperform others or not. What we expect from our bodies and minds as we age, and what we say to ourselves about how we will act as we age, turn out to be powerful predictors.

We can focus on the positives about this time of life: Freedom from worry about others' opinions, hopefully more free time, and wisdom based on our experience. I've been trying out ideas to foster a more positive mindset. See if any of these work for you.

- **Make positive self-affirmations**: When you experience a negative thought about your age, counter it with an equally possible positive idea. If you forget something, remind yourself that your memories are rich. If you notice a wrinkle, remind yourself that wisdom shows on your face. We are strong *and* old. We are beautiful *and* old. We are smart *and* old.
- **Cultivate friendships with age-positive others**: There may be people in your life who are ageist. Counter their

influence by building friendships with age positive people. Make age positive friends at church, in a political action group, in a class, or anywhere you find inspiring, creative and motivated adults. Once you are looking for that vibe, folks who share it will stand out.
- **Connect with organizations that promote positive aging**: There are many options. Websites likeSenior Planet and Old School Clearinghouse, podcasts like Hey Boomer and magazines like Crunchy Tales are just the start.
- **Learn Something New**: Studies show that learning is the best way to keep our minds strong and resilient. Check out OLLI, the Osher Lifelong Learning Institute, for informative classes that have the additional benefit of building connections with others after sixty.
- **Follow Your Passions:** What did you love to do as a child, as a teen, before you took on career and child rearing? What other passions did you set aside for later, during the busy middle of life? Well, later is now. Whether it's cooking, painting, or collecting toy dinosaurs, this is your moment.
- **Do good in the world**: Find a cause that you believe in and a way to help others. There is no better way to demonstrate our worth, including to ourselves. When we contribute to the well-being of others we expand our sense of emotional connection and joy in living.

Recognizing our biases and pushing back on them is the foundation to build age-positive networks. As we practice our own creativity, we create more age-positive stories and art. We can strengthen the culture to benefit ourselves, our peers, and crones in training. And speaking of crones, part of the process is choosing the words we want to describe us.

CHAPTER 4
BY ANY OTHER NAME

When I write about life after midlife, one challenge is just what to call our cohort of women. I've looked at how other authors name us and found no consensus. "Juicy Crones," "Wise Women," "Women Past Midlife," "Women Growing Bolder," "Ripe Women," "Ageless," "Seasoned Women," all have their adherents. There must be fifty ways to avoid saying "older."

This echoes a name challenge our family faced years ago. My son who has cerebral palsy and rides a wheelchair is in his forties now. When he was a child, the California state agency that helped our family was still called "Crippled Children's Services." By then the word "crippled" was already out of favor. The agency soon changed its name to "California Children's Services;" apparently they wished to keep their monogram. Around that time the word "handicapped" came into vogue. Next decade the favored word was "disabled." And then came "differently abled," at which point my son and his friends decided reality had left the building and just started calling each other Crips. Personally, I favor "inconvenienced," but I don't get a vote on this one—at least, not yet, since I am still "temporarily able-bodied."

The issue is not with words themselves. There is nothing inherently good or bad about any word for a woman over fifty, or any word for a person with movement challenges, or anyone in any other group. Rather, words absorb the attitudes of those who use them and take on stigma in people's minds. If you read *Stranger in a Strange Land*, that science fiction classic of the 1960s, you may remember that the Martians in the story abandoned their cities every few centuries and built new ones because the old cities became laden with emotion. Some words become as burdened as an old Martian city.

Combining words with different valences is one way to shake up assumptions. When my friend Lynx Canon began her monthly erotic reading series for women over fifty, she named it "Dirty Old Women," a play on ageism and sexism. When I formed the first "Elderotica" writing group in California, the women appreciated the mashup of "erotica" and "elder."

A word is a nexus of power, and one way we claim our power is by taking ownership of names. Sometimes stigmatized groups reclaim negative terms and use them to push back; think of the Fat Liberation Movement. Sometimes groups lay claim to words with cultural significance, as when queer folk claim the word "gay," which Gertrude Stein used in a story published in 1920: "Helen Furr and Georgine Skeen, they were regularly gay there, where they were gay. To be regularly gay was to do every day the gay thing that they did every day."

By now, we women over fifty – we old broads – have an assortment of names to choose from. Personally, I like "crone," though it originally meant a feeble old woman, or worse yet, carrion. "Crone" has been given a new meaning of crown, or wise woman, who sees so much that the future loses its mystery.

What would your choice be? What words do you hate, or love—and why?

CHAPTER 5
POWER PROFILE
ASHTON APPLEWHITE

> *Aging is a natural, lifelong, powerful process that unites us all. So how come so many of us unthinkingly assume that depression, diapers, and dementia lie ahead? Because of ageism — stereotypes (how we think), prejudice (how we feel), and discrimination (how we act) towards others or ourselves based on age.*
>
> —Ashton Applewhite

Ashton is the first to say she's never had much of a career plan. She never expected to become a writer, let alone a public figure, and didn't start writing until she was in her forties. In 1992 the launch of Ashton's first serious book, *Cutting Loose: Why Women Who End Their Marriages Do So Well*, landed her on Phyllis Schlafly's Enemies List—quite the honor. As Ashton wrote, "The catalyst for *Cutting Loose* was puzzlement: Why was our notion of women's lives after divorce (visualize depressed dame on barstool) so different from the happy and energized reality?"

That same impulse to challenge misleading stereotypes motivated Ashton to start blogging about aging and ageism in 2005, and to write her best-known book, *This Chair Rocks: A Manifesto Against Ageism*. Once again Ashton challenged the dominant narrative: this time the grim portrayal of late life that simply does not match the lives we live. Ashton went on to create a Q&A blog, *Yo! Is this Ageist?* and to establish herself as a public speaker. She received a standing ovation for her 2017 TED talk, which has now been viewed over two million times. In 2022 the United Nations named Ashton one of the Healthy Aging 50: fifty leaders transforming the world to be a better place to grow older.

Ashton is also a co-creator of the Old School Hub, which educates people about ageism and connects people working to end it. Old School hosts a weekly open discussion called Office Hours, and you can almost always find Ashton there. As she says, "Our goal is to help create a world where everyone has the opportunity to live long and to live well."

Ashton believes that all forms of discrimination are linked. She writes:

"We can't dismantle ageism without dismantling ableism—and racism and sexism and homophobia and all the rest—because these are systems of oppression that feed and depend on each other.

- *Age equity requires gender equity, because our systems make aging harder for women.*
- *Age equity requires disability equity, because fears of impairment feed stigma and age shame, and because some impairment awaits us all.*

- *Age equity requires racial equity, because racism denies multitudes the chance to age."*

Ashton is now at work on an initiative called YODA, for "Young and Old Dismantling Ageism," to bring all ages together to talk about power. She hopes this project will derail old vs. young framing, identify shared barriers and goals, and help build a movement for age equity that represents—and outlives—us all.

PART TWO
CREATIVITY

In our sixties, many of us have the time to create that we lacked for much of adult life. It's as if we acquire an artistic patron when we leave full-time employment and our children fly from the nest. Plus, studies have shown that our brains develop new interconnections after sixty that foster our creativity. We can return to the kinds of creative play we enjoyed as children or develop new interests—it's our choice.

Less talked about but just as important: When we express ourselves creatively we counter ageist stereotypes by making it clear we live vivid lives. Plus there are many ways to connect with others with shared creative interests, adding juice to our creativity, and to our social lives.

The essays in this section explore the joys and mischiefs of creating in our sixties.

CHAPTER 6
WHY A DEBUT NOVEL AT AGE 68?

As a book-devouring kid, I planned to write my first novel by age 25. Given that I was not independently wealthy and had what my mother called "champagne taste on a beer budget," that plan was a bit naïve.

Instead, age 25 found me in New York, on my way to an MBA and a rather dry job in finance. Several kids and a divorce later, I earned an MS in biology and switched to a career as a biotech writer. You won't find my name on any books from that era. My work product from that thirty-year stint resides in file drawers at FDA, valuable to my employers but entirely confidential.

Fast forward to age 57, a second divorce, the children mostly grown and fledged, and suddenly I was a late bloomer with an active dating life. Let's just say that after sixty you must kiss a lot of frogs to find a prince. But find him I did, when I was 62 and he was 64. By then I had plenty of stories to tell about love, motherhood, careers, and life in general. Then two things happened in quick succession.

First, I read an article by a well-meaning Romance novelist in her fifties advising her sisters that if they wanted to be published they should write characters in their twenties. Unbelievable! Shades of the Bronte sisters forced to use male pen names. Why should Women Writers of a Certain Age be closeted? I was ticked.

Second, a friend who writes erotica started a monthly reading series at a local bookstore. "Dirty Old Women" showcased the sexy stories of women over fifty. Was I ready to return to my plan to write fiction, a few decades late? Absolutely.

Writing erotica about older women is incredibly liberating. It pushes back on the gendered ageism endemic to our culture with a fun revolution. Reading before a mixed age audience, I was gratified when younger women approached us at the end of the evening to thank us for showing that the sensual side of a woman's life does not end on her fortieth birthday.

That experience led me to start a writing group called Elderotica, with the goal of bringing the joy of sensual writing to other women. That in turn led to my first book, *Aphrodite's Pen: The Power of Writing Erotica after Midlife*. *Pen* includes writing prompts, interviews with older women writers, and examples of their fiction. During the pandemic I wrote stories about women in a locked down retirement community and their (safely paranormal) lovers (*The Erotic Pandemic Collection*).

But I was way overdue to write my first novel. After my story collection launched I finally began that project. *Brilliant Charming Bastard*, published in 2021, is the story of three women scientists in their sixties who discover they are dating the same lying dilettante who is stealing their ideas for his invention. When the women find each other, they form a startup company and outfox their cheating manfriend. The book was great fun to write, not least because the trio of seasoned women meet loving partners later in the story.

My sixties were the best part of my life so far, and I'm not alone. You may recall the U-shaped happiness curve from Chapter 1. People tend to be happiest early in life, and then later, when some of their responsibilities fall away. When our children launch, when our careers wind down, we are free to return to the things we most enjoy. We are free to discover new ways to be creative, new ways to give back to others, and new serenity. But in my case, that serenity is balanced by a myriad of projects.

After *Bastard* published, I decided to push the concept of a sexy older woman to the max. How about a 500-year-old? Hence the heroine of *Vampires of a Certain Age*, who owns a blood bank and provides ethically sourced blood to Midwestern vampires. And that novel, a gothic Romance, led to my next book, *Write & Sell a Well-Seasoned Romance*, a soup-to-nuts guide to create, edit, publish and market a Romance novel with older characters (not necessarily 500 years old, though).

Your path may look nothing like mine. Your creativity will take its own shape, which could be anything from needlepoint to sculpture to starting your own printmaking business. Whatever your passion, whatever your creative spark, it is never too late for beginner's mind. It is always time to play at something new.

CHAPTER 7
THE CRONE RENAISSANCE

We begin our lives as scientists and artists, exploring our world and engaging in play. Then the structures at school prepare us for that long stretch of years when we work and care for others. Some of us find creative careers; most of us tamp down our creative passions for decades. That can change with a Renaissance after sixty.

Why Create in Our Sixties?

Why return to creativity? Because being creative is natural to humans. We thrive on it. Thinking outside the box invigorates our brains. We engage with multiple neural pathways that lie fallow when we focus on logic. Creative pursuits reduce stress, whether we engage in music, visual arts, writing, or dance. And, too, creating gives us more energy, more enthusiasm. We find novel ways to solve creative problems, whether we make jewelry or structure the plot of a story.

As we create, we generate our sense of purpose. When we are in flow there is neither time nor reason to question why we are here. Creativity is a force within each of us that adds to the vibrancy of everyday life. Research shows that being creative helps us live longer, healthier, happier lives. And when we combine creativity with movement, such as when we dance, we gain the benefits of both.

Being creative encourages social engagement—another way to enhance health-span and lifespan. Writing groups, artist collectives, or gathering in the hot tub after dance class are all ways to connect with people with similar creative passions.

Can We Be Creative Later in Life? (Hint: Yes!)

You may have heard that creativity is only for the young. Newer research has debunked that misimpression. Harvard Professor Shelley Carson wrote in *Psychology Today* that brain development in our later years makes us *more* suited to creative endeavors. Our brains become less inhibited and more likely to form connections among disparate ideas, which is the basis of creativity. We develop a broader scope of attention, similar to that of highly creative people. Plus we have a wealth of experience to draw upon.

Where to Start?

How to renew creativity? First, remember that creativity is play, and remind your Inner Critic that there is no right or wrong about play. Doing what we enjoy is goalless. Failing at something new is a win. Reassure your Inner Critic she will be consulted if you decide to take the next step and sell a painting or publish a story. Here are some thoughts on where to start:

- **Doodle:** Begin with the easiest thing: Grab a pen and doodle. Doodling engages a part of the brain that triggers creativity. If you'd like, combine doodling with brainstorming and list kinds of creative play you enjoyed as a young child, or during stolen moments in adulthood. Drawing a mindmap (a visual diagram that organizes ideas) is a great way to combine doodling and brainstorming.
- **Write:** Next, try writing. Write anything. Start with a daily writing prompt from a journal, or sign up for prompts on a website. Buy a copy of *Writing Open the Mind* by Andy Couturier and try his playful prompts. Or put a pen and notebook at your bedside and write down your dreams first thing in the morning. You'll be surprised how much you remember after you've done this for a few days!
- **Do Something Different:** Travel to a new place. Dance in your living room. Take a class. Try a new cuisine. Buy a new sex toy. Read a book in a genre you typically avoid. Novelty is the spark for creativity.

What Next?

Keep exploring via one of these avenues:

- **Julia Cameron's books:** Julia has written forty books fostering creativity. Her book, *It's Never Too Late to Begin Again,* focuses on creativity in later life. The book includes a twelve week program designed to reconnect us with our creative lives, using exercises around a series of themes including Wonder, Freedom, Purpose and Joy. For example, in one exercise she asks her readers to write this prompt five times and then complete the sentence differently each time:

If it weren't too late, I'd...

Because (spoiler alert) it isn't too late at all. Our sixties are the exact right time to engage with our dreams and begin something new—or better yet, try several new things and decide which ones to pursue.

(And by the way, after writing forty books Julia Cameron still has an active Inner Critic she's named Nigel, whom she greets with, "Hello, Nigel! What don't you like this time?")

More ideas below:

- **Osher Lifelong Learning Institute:** Sign up for a class that aligns with your creative interests. Drawing, painting, photography—it's all there for you to try. Or sign up for a class at your local bead shop or adult school. Your town's senior center may also offer art or writing classes. Also check with your local college about auditing classes.
- **Spicy Writing:** Writing either Romance or Erotica is a fun and liberating way to celebrate our vivid lives. Check out one of my books on writing (either *Write & Sell a Well-Seasoned Romance*, or *Aphrodite's Pen*) for prompts and inspiration. Check for writing groups in your area, or start your own!

These are just a few of the many ways to give ourselves the gift of creativity in our sixties and beyond. Because so many of us are blessed with long lives and growing freedom, we can return to the creative play we enjoyed as children or try new adventures in imagination. We are once again scientists and artists, ready for a creative Renaissance.

CHAPTER 8
BLOOD AND INK

A Woman of a Certain Age posted on social media that she was obsessed with getting back at her ex from twenty years ago. He had done her wrong and she was still fuming.

"Get therapy," one woman advised. Sounded pricey.

Another chimed in: "Just forget him." Easier said than done.

A third said, "He's not worth the risk of re-engaging." That comment I agreed with. No need for real-life revenge with its attendant messiness. There is a better way.

"Write a revenge novel," was my advice. "Check out *Brilliant Charming Bastard* for ideas." The wronged woman loved that answer and I hope she writes her novel. Plus I hope she reads my novel (I hope you will, too).

In case you have the itch, here are ten steps to get you started on a tale of vengeance that entertains to the max—and gives your readers the catharsis they're looking for.

Step One: Do Nothing

As they say in the Klingon Empire, revenge is a dish best served cold. If your relationship ended fewer than five years ago, put your ideas on the shelf. Time will give you the perspective you need to create a great story.

In the meantime, *Do Nothing* also means: *Don't Throw Anything Away*. It might seem cathartic to delete those emails and ditch that pile of two-faced love letters. But a bigger catharsis is coming your way, and when you're ready to write, you'll need everything about that schmuck that's on paper or in your laptop.

Step Two: Collect Your Materials

Once you have time and distance, start digging. Did you keep a journal back then? Do you have emails in either direction? Letters? Divorce documents? Photos? Pull it together and look for the best nuggets: All the grandiose, self-serving, smarmy language you can find from that self-centered so-and-so. Now make a rough timeline of events and peg your best materials to your timeline.

Step Three: Raise the Stakes

When it comes to revenge, maybe you've thought about slashing his tires or smashing her windshield. That's small potatoes. We're talking fiction now, and anything can happen on the page. Let's raise the stakes: How would you like him to die? Given your history with her, what would be the most ironic, most fitting, dare I say funniest, way you could finish them off?

Only on paper, of course.

Brainstorm ideas. Keep in mind that their death does not necessarily involve murder. Your nasty character could meet their demise solely as a consequence of their own hubris. For example, in *Brilliant Charming Bastard* (spoiler alert), the villain makes a clandestine sex video of the heroine, and after she dumps him, he sits down to watch it and chokes to death on popcorn. Many readers say that's their favorite part of the story.

Next, look at your brainstorm death list, pick your three juiciest ideas and write them up. Have fun with it (Bet you feel better already). Hang onto all three versions of your villain's demise. One version will feature prominently in your novel.

Step Four: Gather Your Posse

Your main character does not need to go it alone. In fact, she should not.

First of all, for whom is she taking revenge? It may be for someone else. For example, in Mindy McGinnis' novel *The Female of the Species*, the heroine, Alex, avenges her sister's death and then branches out to other deserving folks in town.

But beyond her empathy with the victim, a vengeance warrior should always have a posse. Here are some ideas:

- If you're writing from your own experience, consider creating a sidekick character with the wisdom you have now.

- How about modeling a character on friends who gave you good (or bad!) advice back in the day.
- Consider the various aspects of your own personhood: Your Inner Xena, your Inner Femme, your Inner Nerd. To lapse momentarily into psychobabble, a revenge novel can reintegrate the parts of the main character that shattered during trauma (Check out Internal Family Systems Theory, if this concept isn't too Berkeley).

Your main character is not alone in relishing vengeance. Revenge novels get a bad rap, mostly from male reviewers with writer exes. But many women love these stories. Revenge is sweet, and even sweeter when shared. Just think how popular movies like *First Wives' Club* and *The Witches of Eastwick* have been, where a trio of women support one another on their journey to retribution. Those great movies were based on even better revenge novels.

While you develop your posse, make notes on your main characters. That means both your heroine and your villain. (Yes, your villain is a full character too. If they are a cardboard cutout your story will lack spark.) Who are they, and what do they most want? How did their early experiences shape them? What do your characters fear most? What do they look like? Know your characters well enough to convey their *gravitas*: a sense of authority over their own lives. The better you know your characters, the richer a tale you'll tell.

Step Five: Choose Your Settings

This is the perfect time to mention *autofiction*, my favorite strategy for writers over fifty. Autofiction draws on our life history to mix and match places, times, events and people. One of the joys of decades of experience is the many lives we access when we write. We may have travelled, moved cities, worked different jobs. Your novel need not take place in its actual location; in fact, it's better if it does not.

Mixing and matching, whether it's settings or the different attributes of your main characters, moves your story further into fiction. To paraphrase Anne Lamott, if people wanted you to write nicely about them, they shouldn't have been jerks. Yet while the object of your revenge may deserve the worst, writers can land in legal hot water for dissing recognizable people.

So move your story. If it happened when you were teaching school, set it in another part of your life when you worked in a veterinary hospital. Give your villain a career that is different than in real life, more fitting to their nature, in a place that is familiar to you but not to them. Reword those smarmy love letters you saved (but make them just as icky). And of course, change your characters' names.

Step Six: Construct Your Plot
You've already started the process of creating the plot:

- You made a rough timeline of real life events in Step Two
- You raised the stakes with several versions of a villain death scene in Step Three
- You considered how the posse might help resolve the story in Step Four

Choose from the additional ideas below as you assemble your plot:

- Consider ways your story can overturn conventional assumptions about women after midlife. For example, one trope about romance and women after midlife is that women get taken advantage of. And while that can happen, it's certainly not the only outcome of a late-life romance. What if the heroine ruins the villain financially, instead of the other way around? What if your heroine finds a new and better romance after dispatching the villain? Try other counter-tropes: Maybe the heroine is a late bloomer who begins to love sex after fifty. Maybe she wears loud colors, starts lifting weights, or becomes a grey-haired dominatrix. She is, after all, not you, but a fully embodied character who springs from your imaginings (For more on counter-tropes, see my book, *Write & Sell a Well-Seasoned Romance*).

- Next, consider the Heroine's Journey (as distinct from Joseph Campbell's vision of the Hero's Journey). In a revenge novel, the transformation of the heroine can be the main plot driver. What events could you use to show the heroine embracing the masculine side of her character, dealing with her inner conflicts, reconnecting with her feminine side, and becoming a spiritual warrior who celebrates all parts of herself?

- No discussion of plots could omit the famous Three Act Structure that has dominated Western plotting since the Ancient Greeks. Graph it out and the structure looks like sex: Rising action, followed by climax and resolution. Look at the events you have outlined, from life and from your imagination. Capture each event in a few words on a file card, spread out your cards and play with the order. Keeping the Three Act Structure in mind, where in the sequence is each event most satisfying? Where does the villain's death happen in the sequence—in the middle, or closer to the end? And which version of their death best fits your overall story? (And by the way, if you just want your villain humiliated, not actually dead, that's fine too.)

If you're really into planning, you could also write a detailed character arc for each of your main characters and sidekicks. But by now you may be itching to get on with it. Prepare much more and you'll just be procrastinating. Instead, let's write.

Step Seven: Write Your First Draft

Don't try to be measured and mature about your first efforts. Give yourself permission to write complete trash; you need never show this draft to anyone but you. The first draft of a revenge novel can and should be vengeful and petty, on top of the usual failings of any other first draft: cliché-ridden, repetitive, disorganized and incoherent. Write quickly, without editing, and ask your Inner Critic to take a back seat. She can have a turn later.

Have fun with your first draft. Create detailed settings that highlight the motives of your characters. For example, in *Brilliant Charming Bastard*, the appalling state of the villain's refrigerator shows us how he treats women: He serves the fresh food on top to his new conquests and the rotting food underneath to the women he takes for granted.

Step Eight: Do Nothing. Again.

Yes, we are back to a reprise of Step One. Only this time you have a full draft of a revenge novel and can pat yourself on the back about it, even if (especially if) that draft is total garbage.

Congratulate yourself and then stick your draft in a drawer for a month or two or three. Leave your draft alone until you have enough distance to pick out the diamonds amidst the coal.

Step Nine: Edit

Whole books are written on editing, and on its three main phases:

- *Developmental editing*, where you consider what to add and rearrange to make the story even stronger. A writing group can be very handy for this stage.
- *Line editing*, where you polish the language of a story until it sings. Reading aloud will tell you much about the changes needed -- including what to carve away to show off your story. And make sure your dialog includes every witty, caustic comment you didn't think of at the time, but have since!
- *Proofreading*, the last to be done, where you (and your Inner Critic) read the story ten times and are still finding typos.

Pro Tip: Trade proofing sessions with another writer. It's almost impossible to catch every typo in your own work.

Some editing points that are especially relevant to revenge:

- Make sure your villain's comeuppance is supremely satisfying. Look at all three versions of their demise. Are there elements you want to add to the version you chose for your draft?
- Write your heroine at least one great sex scene with a new and better partner after the villain is vanquished. Remember: Anything can happen on the page. And this should happen.
- Revenge can be heavy slogging unless it is balanced by humor. Find ways to add levity to your story. It could be via a foolish sidekick character. It could be narrator

commentary. In the case of *Brilliant Charming Bastard*, a fictional newspaper columnist parodies events in the story.

Step Ten: Share Your Story with the World

Your story is finished, edited, in the best shape you can make it. Now what? Do you need an agent? Maybe not. Check out Duotrope for publishers that accept direct submissions from authors.

Do you even need a publisher? Maybe not that either. The closer you move toward self-publishing, the more time you'll need to put into it AND the more control you will gain. One place to start is my blog series on the publishing process (see the Stella Fosse website). And there's lots more about publishing and marketing in my 2024 book, *Write & Sell a Well-Seasoned Romance*, available at all the online places. Just think of your revenge novel as an anti-Romance.

Whether or not you decide to publish, you've now written your revenge novel, created your alternate universe, and given yourself, and potentially others, a vision of rough justice. You have performed an exorcism, and you will be stronger for it.

Stories are powerful and to be a teller of tales is a significant responsibility. It is also a significant joy. May you revel in your tale of revenge.

CHAPTER 9
THE UNFETTERED BLISS OF TRYING SOMETHING NEW

Creating in familiar ways leads to certain expectations. Our Inner Critic has particular standards for what we do on the regular. I'm always looking for ways to sidestep her. I found the perfect method to circumvent the Critic years ago, when I was invited to Sanctuary, a Bay Area retreat hosted by my friend Susan Ito, author of the award-winning memoir *I Would Meet You Anywhere*.

Susan first discovered the Santa Sabina Retreat Center when she attended a calligraphy workshop there. She fell in love with the place. No wonder. Santa Sabina was once a novitiate, a home for nuns in training. Built with monastic rooms around a lush central courtyard, the Center invites us to gaze inward. After several solo writing retreats, Susan decided to host annual gatherings at Santa Sabina every New Year.

Susan is an artist as well as a writer and invites friends of both persuasions to her retreats. She provides an array of supplies including mountains of collage materials as well as calligraphy pens and inks. Magic happens in that sacred space because *the artists write and the writers make art.*

I attended Sanctuary on and off for a dozen years. And in the same way that some folks convince themselves that they are "not writers," before Sanctuary I was sure I was no artist. For all my preaching about the importance of play, and how essential it is to set aside negative judgement about first drafts, I had never examined my own aversion to anything artistic. But those collage supplies were so tempting. And here is what I discovered: *There is no such thing as a bad collage* (just like there is no such thing as a bad first draft).

The process of looking through materials, finding images that appeal (for whatever reason), of cutting them out and trying different arrangements on the page, is contemplative and satisfying in ways I cannot explain. The final product almost always looks great. And if it doesn't, a collage can just be cut into strips and woven into another collage.

In my first effort, a monster's head tops the torso of a woman pirate in full regalia. Next to her a cutout of a Rumi poem admonishes us to marry the ocean the first chance we get. I was instantly bitten by the collage bug, and soon had my own stack of catalogs and calendars. My first pandemic collage features a woman whose head is encased in a glass dome. I made many others, including a Rube Goldberg montage in which a tiny hammer sets off a cascade of improbable events that finally ends in a broken lightbulb. Collages decorate my house and some I've sent off as gifts. Over the years I've hosted collage parties at home, where my friends can discover this amazing process for themselves. So can you.

You may already have some materials at home, and collecting them is easy. Save old wall calendars, along with bits of ribbon and the best of the clothing catalogs that arrive in the mail (Gudren Sjoden features models past midlife). *American Showcase* is an annual illustration catalog with high quality examples from a variety of graphic artists, and the out-of-date volumes are inexpensive online. For backing use watercolor paper or whatever is on hand; Susan buys unused pizza boxes from pizzerias for three-dimensional collages that also store unused cutouts. Use glue sticks to join up your images. Once they are dry, burnish with Mod Podge for an integrated look. Collaging goes beyond easy and fun. It's not a stretch to call it a spiritual practice.

To host your own collage party, ask everyone to bring a pair of scissors and a magazine or catalog. Have plenty of paper and glue sticks on hand, plus several *American Showcase* catalogs. Choose a simple theme or prompts if you would like, or go free-form. Encourage everyone to share or swap materials, explain the basics and have a great time.

I truly believe that we are all writers. Collage teaches another lesson: *We are all artists.* And one more truth to bear in mind: *Every one of us deserves to play.*

CHAPTER 10
CREATIVITY PROFILE
JAKI SHELTON GREEN

I find that many women are practicing ancestor worship but passing by those of us who are still here. We must repossess the agency of the Crone. We must not allow others to set it aside.

—Jaki Shelton Green

Jaki Shelton Green is the first African American and the third woman to be named Poet Laureate of North Carolina. Her poetry celebrates the mythmaking South, mourns and honors the life of her daughter, and is by turns angry and wickedly funny. She says, "Becoming Poet Laureate is a big deal for a brown girl from Efland, North Carolina. I have sat at tables where my grandmother would have been serving. My ancestors have been in those rooms, but not as guests, and certainly not as celebrity guests. It comes with a responsibility to give back, to nurture."

In her fifties, Green left her job as Director of a non-profit to write and teach writing full time. Initially she was terrified. "I did not know what it meant to be the writer." Over time she published multiple books of poetry, and her work has been featured in translations and videos. She has earned many honors besides her Poet Laureate status, and leads classes that transform the lives of women who want to be creative but are held back by internal bias. She hosts writing retreats for women in many locations across the United States and in Morocco.

Green focuses on women's responsibility to support one another across generations. "When I was a child, my mother and her friends would take cuttings from one another's yards. My grandmother grew peonies from cuttings. Once I was in a swimming pool and an older woman recognized me and told me she had a yard full of peonies grown from a cutting from my grandmother's yard. The question is, what do we as older women have to offer one another? How about a Cronefest, a moveable feast, where we take turns hosting a Sunday brunch? How about one woman could be another's Blue Apron and prepare her dinners for two weeks? How about we create our own Crone Currency that we could use with each other?"

Green firmly believes in the agency of the Crone. "What advice do I have for women wanting to pursue creativity after sixty? Get out of your own way. Find out what is stopping you. Who is tying your feet to the ground? What are you afraid of? And what will happen to you if you *don't* do it?"

PART THREE
SEXUALITY

The sexuality of women over forty—much less sixty—is often ignored or ridiculed by society. Yet sexuality and sensuality are innate traits that belong to each woman, just like her laugh and her eye color. The essays in this section explore and celebrate this essential aspect of life after sixty.

PART THREE
SEXUALITY

CHAPTER 11
PASSION ABIDES

I was a Late Bloomer when it came to the erotic side of life. And I'm not alone – there is a whole subgenre of erotic romance about women like me.

So there I was, arriving at the party when most everyone was packing up to leave. I was just divorced at 57 and there was this new thing called online dating. What liberation, compared with my mother's generation of divorced ladies.

Some people say that dating online after 50 is like looking through a yard sale for the one dusty object you wouldn't mind taking home. Others use my favorite metaphor: you have to kiss a lot of frogs to find a prince. No matter how you phrase it, online dating takes persistence and a sense of humor.

First there was the shock of sitting across a café table from some guy with white hair. What happened to the boys of my youth? That was easy: While I wasn't looking, they turned into guys with white hair.

Then there was the fellow who looked like a professor, patches at the elbows of his tweed jacket, who finished his dinner and said, "While I can't pay for my meal, if you pay for us both, I will gladly gift you a copy of my novel."

And then there was the gent who insisted he was monogamous. It turned out he said that to all the ladies—even the ones in open marriages who couldn't have cared less.

Was it all worth it? Absolutely. I discovered so much about the passionate side of life that I had suspected existed but never really known. I had my heart broken, sure, but I also learned a lot.

I learned that erotic bliss has no time limit. Society tries to sexualize girls way too young, and then tries to unsex women before we are ready. But the reality is that passion abides.

I learned that there are physical changes to manage such as Genitourinary Syndrome of Menopause (GSM). Thinning of the membranes in the vulva and vagina can lead to dryness, frequent urination, and discomfort during intercourse. GSM affects more than half of women after sixty. You would expect to hear a lot about it, like the changes at puberty we talked about so much when we were young. But GSM is seldom discussed, which may be one reason pharmaceutical companies were able to overprice the treatment for so long. A topical estrogen cream that costs about the same to manufacture as toothpaste retailed for decades at hundreds of dollars a tube.

I learned from my own body: what brings me bliss, and how that changes over time. What I enjoyed in my late 60s was different than in my 50s, but the feelings are just as strong.

I learned from books, like Joan Price's terrific *Naked at Our Age*, a guide to continued sexual joy as our bodies change.

I learned what it's like to be an adventurer at 60, and then over the last decade, I've learned what it is to have a loving sexy life companion. Is it late to be learning that? Who cares? Some people never get to have what I have now. I am also learning that most important life lesson, gratitude.

One source of gratitude is my network of women friends, especially a group called Elderotica that has been writing together for a dozen years. This circle of women shared discoveries about sexuality and sensuality in our sixties as we wrote together, laughed together, chatted and snacked. We also published an anthology of our stories, but our value as friends goes far beyond our writing life.

As each woman reaches her sixties, she makes her own decisions about the decade ahead. Some of us are grateful to leave sexuality behind after menopause, to focus on different aspects of learning and growth. Other women continue our sex lives unabated, and still others are late bloomers who fully connect with sexuality and sensuality after the children have grown and career demands lighten. And, too, women who experienced sexual abuse in their youth may need decades to heal to the point where they can fully engage sexually. When they arrive at that level of healing, cultural messages may say it's too late, their sexual lives are over. Those messages are simply not true. As

STELLA FOSSE

Virginia Woolf said, "The older one gets, the more one likes indecency."

Whatever path you take after sixty, however you choose to express your vibrant nature, may your later life be full of new learning, new connections, and new joys.

CHAPTER 12
SEXUAL AGENCY AFTER SIXTY

We are born to be creative and sensual. Our bodies are ours and our sexuality is ours. Although women of every age are objectified in American culture, our sexuality is innate. And sex after sixty is good for us. Studies show that it improves heart health, lowers stress, and promotes our well-being in other ways, from decreased pain to better sleep. Yet our culture denigrates the sexuality of older women and too often objectifies young girls.

In her 2016 book, *Girls and Sex: Navigating the Complicated New Landscape*, Peggy Orenstein describes the pressure on American women to perform sexually from an early age—and to please young men while doing so. Sadly their own pleasure is too often not the focus of how young women view sex. How sexuality is portrayed in the media and online contributes to this problem. Studies show that movie and television executives choose to portray males as active and females as passive, even in Saturday morning cartoons for children. And because of the internet, young people today are exposed to pornographic images that normalize aggressive sexual behavior. As an antidote, Orenstein recommends parents take the lead in discussing with girls the importance of their own desires, highlighting the girls' power and agency.

For women who did not have that kind of mentoring and family support, it can take years or decades to overcome social suppression of sexual agency. And for women who have experienced sexual aggression, healing can take half a lifetime. By the time a woman becomes comfortable with her sexuality and fully owns her desires, her sexuality as a midlife woman is downplayed by society. The sexuality of older women is frequently ignored or reviled in Western culture. From the British program "How Not to Get Old" (which offers "beauty" treatments so extreme that one reviewer said "Die young. That's the only sensible solution,") to the negative examples of powerful but evil older female Disney villains, the erotic power of women past menopause is stigmatized rather than celebrated.

The good news is that we are seeing a shift in media portrayals. Emma Thompson's 2022 movie, *Good Luck to You, Leo Grande*, is an intimate portrait of a woman in her sixties claiming her pleasure for the first time. And the advent of the "Seasoned Romance" enables older writers to publish stories about characters their own age, instead of camouflaging their hard-won erotic knowledge in characters in their twenties.

For women of every age—younger women pushed into sexual behavior, and midlife women discouraged from claiming their sexuality—the central issue is ownership of our erotic power. Paying attention to their own pleasure is essential for young women, and it is just as essential for women past midlife.

So how do we navigate the sensual landscape of our later years? We can start by paying attention to what brings us joy. How we respond to music, stars, trees and birds is something each of us owns. We also own our enjoyment of sexual play, whether partnered or not. Delight is our guide as we seek out positive portrayals of ripe sexy women in books, movies, and online. The women creating this material deserve our support, and we deserve to be lifted up by their art. From famous writers like Erica Jong (*Fear of Dying*) to less well known but excellent writers like Rae Padilla Francoeur (*Free Fall: A Late-in-Life Love Affair*), women are creating a shared erotic narrative that continues for a lifetime.

We begin life with freedom to play and create. We can give ourselves the gift of returning to that creative place after midlife. For every positive story that has been written about women after sixty, there are hundreds left to tell. For every photograph taken of a beautiful older face, there are hundreds left to capture. Paying attention to our own joy, choosing to read positive stories, and creating for ourselves, are some of the many pathways to claiming our bliss.

CHAPTER 13
THE NITTY GRITTY

It's all well and good to say that sexuality is our birthright, but how to maintain that birthright after sixty? The first step is to celebrate the sensual aspect of life each day. Give yourself a facial. Dance to your favorite song. Soak in a scented tub.

Because giving ourselves pleasure is key. After all, a woman's closest and most reliable sexual partner is herself. Masturbation warrior Betty Dodson was a sexual pioneer who believed that in order to be truly equal, women must be independent from men for their sexual satisfaction. She is famous for her trailblazing work empowering women through masturbation, including her many hands-on workshops and her book, *Sex for One*.

The quest for the perfect vibrator for older women made a big splash in the television show *Grace and Frankie* in 2017. In the show, the two main characters create and market a sex toy aptly named "Menage a Moi." How lovely that a television show focused on postmenopausal women developing a sex toy. This imaginary toy had lots of helpful features: glow-in-the-dark controls, light weight, and a soft grip gel sleeve.

Joan Price, who writes extensively about senior sexuality, points out that real toys can have even more features than the fictional "Menage a Moi." These include rechargeable batteries, multiple vibration settings, and being waterproof for use in the tub or shower. Safe materials are important; if you look for a new toy, it is a good idea to check for a CE mark, which indicates the product meets European safety standards.

When it comes to sex toys, standard vibrators are not the whole story. Toys with suction can be a great addition to the toy bag of the sexy older woman. These toys, called "air pulse" or "clitoral suction" vibrators, provide a very different sensation that is out of keeping with their appearance (which is something like a banana slug with one end cut off). And last but not least, be sure to choose lubricants that promote enjoyment, whether having sex solo or with a partner. While lube is great at any time in life, it is especially helpful after menopause. Lubricants differ. Silicone lube may be gentler for sensitive older genitals (although not advised when using a silicone sex toy). The moisturizing effects of lubricants with aloe vera can be helpful (unless you're allergic). Certain ingredients, such as glycerin and petroleum jelly, are best avoided to minimize the risk of a urinary tract or vaginal infection.

Reclaiming Sexuality after Trauma

Sexual abuse early in life can affect our sexual enjoyment for decades. And people who have been abused may be discouraged from speaking the truth of what happened, may even find it difficult to acknowledge to themselves. What we saw during the #metoo movement was the beginning of survivors finding a collective voice. Yet stories of incest were rare; perhaps the voices of incest survivors are even harder to hear. And yet we know that finding our voice is a powerful part of reclaiming our sexual joy.

In her book, *Writing Ourselves Whole: Using the Power of Your Own Creativity to Recover and Heal from Sexual Trauma,* author Jen Cross describes her experience leading writing groups for trauma survivors. When people write their stories of abuse, they break the silence they carry and acknowledge each other as creative beings. Writing freely, as a practice over time, has the power to transform us, to bring us back to our desires.

Many women who are survivors, who have worked through trauma for decades, come home to our bodies after midlife. Although we are changed by our experiences, we reclaim our agency. We mourn the years we lost, but rejoice in the freedom to begin again. And when we gain that freedom, the women of our generation who are "late bloomers" are lucky to have more opportunities to find romantic and sexual partners than did survivors in the past.

Finding a Partner after Midlife

As Laura Stassi says in her book *Romance Redux,* there are three main ways to meet new people after midlife:

- In real life, through doing things you love, like taking a class or going to church
- By reviving connections with someone you knew in your youth

- Through an online dating service

Meeting someone in real life has big advantages. You come to know the person gradually as friends, so that you know who you are dealing with before a friendship becomes a romance. And if you are doing something you love to do, the time is well spent whether you meet someone or not.

Reconnecting with someone from decades ago is more common now in the age of the internet. There were always high school and college reunions, but with the proliferation of social media, more of us are connecting with friends and former lovers we have not seen in decades. We revive connections, and sometimes romances, with people we knew long ago.

But the biggest change in the dating lives of women after midlife is the advent of online dating, a source of many possibilities, both good and not so good. We often hear cautionary tales about women scammed by people who claim to have fallen in love and who prey on women's wishes to find a partner. All the common sense rules apply: Meet in a public place. Get to know the person well before giving personal information, getting into a car with them, going to their home or inviting them to yours. Never give money to someone you're dating. Even those who are not overt scammers may misrepresent their background or their intentions. And just as in everyday life, some on these sites harbor prejudice against older women, women of size, women of color. Online dating requires a skeptical nature and a tough skin.

We hear less about the online success stories: older women meeting real people online who are well intentioned and honest about what they seek, whether that be a long-term relationship or a one-night stand; a monogamous or polyamorous arrangement; and whether they are gay, straight or bisexual. Understand your own goals so that you can find potential partners who are sympatico, with the knowledge that what you want (and what others want) can change over time.

Ageism in Dating

To be comfortable with dating after sixty requires that we do as much as we can to heal our Inner Ageist. We may think we have a rapport with our bodies, but what comes up when we allow a new lover to see our breasts, our bellies, as they are now? And when we meet someone new and begin to cultivate physical intimacy, how will we feel about the evidence of age on that person's physique? Prepare ahead of time. Appreciate your own naked body, tell yourself what you like about it. And when the time comes, look for what you like about your new lover's body. They have swum in the cultural ageist soup all their lives too. Tell them what appeals to you about what you see.

Sexual Expression in Long-Term Relationships

Relationships meet our needs for security and for passionate connection—two powerful human drives that are somewhat contradictory. When we first connect with a prospective partner, passion is foremost. The unknown is captivating; it spurs us to explore, to connect. Fast forward past twenty or forty years of domestic life and novelty has largely been replaced by security. Our long-time partners are well known to us. We know how kind they are, how steadfast, and we also know their habits, their bodily functions, and their foibles.

In her book, *Mating in Captivity*, psychologist Esther Perel explains that to maintain passion in a long-term relationship requires us to see our partners as if they were new to us. This may mean sitting in the audience when they give a talk, observing how engaged others are in what our lover has to say. Or it may require spending the occasional week or weekend apart, coming together again to talk about our adventures.

Those of us in long-term relationships are in them for a reason. Something about the other person entices us. Underneath the domestic routines of days and years, that extraordinary human being is with us, still present, still sexy. We can rediscover their sublime nature and keep our passion alive.

Older Lesbians

Like all of us now in our sixties and seventies, older Lesbians grew up in a time when sexual behavior by unmarried women was shamed and shunned. In addition to that socialization, Lesbians of our generation came of age soon after the Stonewall uprising, when Lesbianism was still seen as the result of mental health issues. Many Lesbians now in their sixties and seventies were caretakers for gay men with AIDS. Many were part of the movement to extend marriage rights to LGTBQ+ Americans. Pride in Lesbian identity has roots in a long struggle. For these women, many of whom maintain close and loving relationships for decades, novelty and separateness can be important. Making a sex date and anticipating the joy ahead, adding toys and edible fruit lotions to sex play, and beginning with slow dancing can all add romance to the occasion.

Choices After Sixty

It is no secret that there are more women than men after sixty. That discrepancy grows larger the longer we live. For those of us whose history is heterosexual and monogamous, finding a partner after sixty may require creative choices. Which approach works best is different for different women, and for each of us over time. Two traits can be especially helpful.

- **Perseverance**: As I've said before, in later life you must kiss a lot of frogs to find a prince. But kissing frogs can be fun, especially if you only kiss the ones with prince potential.
- **Curiosity**: Date someone outside your comfort zone to find out where your comfort zone really is. Perhaps you wonder whether you might be bisexual. Consider dating women and see what that experience is like. Perhaps you are curious about polyamory and are ready to date someone in an open relationship. If your career is or was professional, you might try dating a tradesperson (or vice versa). Dating someone unexpected can bring much novelty to a romance.

Conclusion

Women live longer than ever and have more choices than ever. After age sixty we have outlived the possibility of pregnancy and, for most of us, the children are grown and fledged. Whether we have long been sexually engaged or are blooming into sexual life, sensuality and sexuality can be a fabulous part of our juicy lives after sixty—especially if we pay attention to the nitty gritty.

CHAPTER 14
TOP TEN REASONS WHY WOMEN OVER SIXTY SHOULD WRITE EROTICA

Ever since I wrote *Aphrodite's Pen: The Power of Writing Erotica after Midlife*, older women who don't write erotica have asked me to break it down. In essence, the question is "What's in it for me?" Here are my top ten reasons.

1. Writing erotica is liberating. Any time we write, we play ruler of the universe. When we write erotica, we play Sex Goddess. We capture our fondest erotic memories and write fiction about our desires. Nothing is more freeing than this kind of creative play.

2. Writing erotica is fun. We can be as playful as we want; there is no need to judge ourselves. Remember the dreaded Five Paragraph Essay in high school? This is **nothing** like that. Writing erotica is pure play, a journey through memories and might-have-beens. No judgement, no second guessing, only delight.

3. Writing erotica is a great way to express and empower ourselves. Even when we write for our own enjoyment, even if you never show what you write to another soul, your own erotica will bring you joy. It connects you with wishes and memories as nothing else can. Going back and revisiting our own erotica is a wonderful way to bring back the details of precious moments and fantasies.

4. Older women have a store of experience to draw upon as we create story. At our age we possess a deep understanding of human nature. We understand the desires and foibles of women and men, we know how conflict arises and how it resolves. This wisdom runs deeper than memory and informs all we write.

5. Starting an **erotic writing group** is a great way to encourage and empower each other and to build a community of writers. Older women who write erotica are fun and creative mutineers. They are some of the most engaging people I know. Writing erotica together and sharing it is so fun that it must be experienced.

6. Writing erotica turns society's expectations about older women upside down. This is a good thing. When we write about women who are confident in the sexiness of our older selves, we create a healthy alternative narrative about older women that is much needed.

7. If we decide to share our writing, we let younger women know that there is joy ahead, and that our erotic lives **can** continue into our sixties, seventies, and beyond. When I read sexy stories to a mixed age audience, many younger women are relieved to hear that a woman's erotic life does not stop at forty. The scarcity of older erotic

role models in popular culture makes young people anxious. We can help.

8. Plenty of women and men want to hear about us as we really are. Historically, it was easier to publish erotica if you were writing younger characters. The more women over fifty who write erotica, the more of us who publish erotica, and the more readers engage with what we write, the more these outmoded barriers break down.

9. There could (and should) be more women of age writing sexy stories. Some older women are writing and publishing erotica – like Erica Jong's *Fear of Dying*, or Joan Price's anthology, *Ageless Erotica*. Published Elderotica can be great inspiration for new writing. Check out *Free Fall* by Rae Padilla Francoeur, or Sharon Olds' poems in *Odes*. There are more examples on the Stella Fosse website. But more voices are needed – including yours.

10. "Why erotica at this time of life? Why not? We're not dead yet." This quote is from my friend Billie Berlin. All I can say is Amen, sister. As the saying goes, "If not now, when? And if not us, who?"

CHAPTER 15
SEXUALITY PROFILE
JOAN PRICE

*It's **not too late** to embrace a different version of sexuality that fits your needs now, even if it conflicts with what you were taught decades ago. You've let go of other beliefs and restrictions that no longer serve you. Examine your convictions about sex and relationships with an open mind.*

—Joan Price

Joan Price began her work on sexuality for olders after 22 years as an English teacher and a career as a health and fitness writer. She fell in love at age 57 and enjoyed a passionate relationship with Robert Rice, who was then 64. Joan's first book about senior sex, *Better Than I Ever Expected: Straight Talk about Sex After Sixty*, prompted many questions from readers about their sexual challenges. Her award-winning next book, *Naked at Our Age*, looks at how to continue enjoying sexuality despite the challenges of an aging body. Joan continued her work as a "senior sexpert" after her husband Robert's death, giving talks, writing an advice column for *Senior Planet,* and reviewing sex toys on her website.

A decade after Robert's passing, Joan felt ready to publish a book about sexuality after the death of a partner. *Sex after Grief: Navigating Your Sexuality after Losing Your Beloved* is her gift to women and men recovering from loss.

In addition to her nonfiction books, Joan edited a story anthology called *Ageless Erotica* that was published in 2013. She collected these stories because, as she wrote, "my aging brain wants to be stimulated by sexy stories that reflect my experience and the realities of my age group in a way that's both truthful and racy. I neither wish nor need to go back in time to spark my fire, even in my fantasies."

In between international speaking engagements, Joan continues her interest in fitness. Now in her eighties, she teaches line dancing in her home town of Sebastopol, California.

Learn more about Joan Price and her work at her website (https://joanprice.com) and follow her column on *Senior Planet.*

PART FOUR
HEALTHCARE

Actively managing our health is an important part of self-care after sixty. Although most healthcare expenses (and most of the profits for the healthcare industry) come from people over sixty, research is lacking about our age group for everything from defining normal lab results to determining which treatments are effective. Older women may encounter doctors who dismiss their symptoms, while other doctors over-diagnose, overprescribe and over-treat.

Every treatment has risks and benefits; only you can decide what is right for you. As they say, fortune favors the prepared mind. The essays in this section focus on healthcare strategies for our sixties and beyond.

CHAPTER 16
MANAGE YOUR HEALTHCARE

When my mother trained in the Cadet Nursing Corps during World War II, young nurses were taught that physicians could do no wrong. Yet if a doctor did make a mistake, it was the nurses' duty to cover for the doctor. When I was a child, Mom worked in the obstetrics ward of our local hospital and came home with stories of doctors who stayed too long on the golf course when called to a difficult birth, or mishandled forceps and damaged a baby during delivery. Nevertheless, as a young woman I shared the common belief that doctors were demigods whose judgement should not be questioned.

Over time I came to realize that physicians are just as fallible as anyone else. Physicians are trained in a set of objective problem-solving tools but bring unconscious bias to their work. As a woman, I have experienced the sexism inherent in medicine. As the mother of a disabled adult, I've witnessed ableism in healthcare. Weightism in clinical care is well documented. And as a biotechnology professional I saw evidence that clinical research is biased in favor of whites.

Studies show that, on average, older people are taken less seriously than younger people when they report disease symptoms. These issues are compounded for older women who face gendered medical ageism. For women of color and women with disabilities, the challenges are even greater.

While many physicians are highly competent and provide excellent care, consider these suggestions to prevent or push back on medical ageism.

- Make a list ahead of seeing your doctor that includes relevant history and your questions/concerns. Bring two copies to your appointment, one for you and one for the physician. Ensure you get answers to all your points. (See the Summary Sheet in Step 3, below.)
- Take notes and ask follow-up questions.
- If an issue is not dealt with, use an "I statement," as in: "I feel my concern has not been addressed fully. Let's circle back to _____." If a physician dismisses your concerns, ask them to use their professional skills to work with you and find a solution.
- Consider bringing someone with you for support. That person can confirm, for example, that the level of pain you are experiencing is unusual. But if the healthcare professional interacts with your support person instead of you, remind the physician that you are the patient and are there to ask and answer questions.
- If a medical person addresses you in a condescending way (for example calling you "young lady") let them know that, while you understand they mean no harm, you prefer to be addressed by your name. Remind them that you are Ms. ____.
- If a physician is not providing adequate care, find a different one. You deserve excellent care.

Here is the process I've developed to foster a team approach on my medical visits. Please use what suits your needs.

Step 1: Self-Education

Before visiting a physician about a health issue, consult reputable sources to learn about your concern. Look for information on:

- What causes the condition?
- What are common symptoms?
- What are treatment options for this health issue, including pluses and minuses of each?
- What is the prognosis?
- What can I do at home to lessen the impact of this medical issue?

Some physicians complain about patients who consult "Dr. Google" before coming to see them. However, recent studies have shown that when patients inform themselves by reading *reliable* online materials, their interactions with healthcare professionals are more productive. Sources like the Mayo Clinic and the *Journal of the American Medical Society* are helpful. On the other hand, AI-based tools like ChatGPT or Google Gemini have high rates of inaccuracy for medical advice and should be avoided.

Step 2: In God We Trust, All Others Bring Data

Not every health complaint can be documented by home data. But when it is possible to bring data to a medical visit, that's a great way to focus the doctor's attention on the issue at hand. Here are examples of ways to collect data:

- **Apple Watch**: Your watch can collect data about atrial fibrillation, heart rate at rest and in motion, and blood oxygen. All this data can be exported, shared with your doctor, or printed to bring to an appointment.
- **O_2 Meter**: This is an inexpensive device that slips over the finger and measures the level of oxygen in the blood. Many people purchased these during the COVID pandemic, and they remain a reliable way of determining whether a respiratory infection is interfering with oxygen levels.
- **Blood Pressure Cuff**: If you, as I do, have "White Coat Syndrome" and your blood pressure goes up the minute you walk into the doctor's office, take your blood pressure at home in the morning before your visit and photograph the results. Encourage medical staff to wait at least five minutes from the time you sit down in the exam room before taking your blood pressure. If blood pressure is not the issue you want to discuss, don't allow your appointment to veer off in an unproductive direction.

Some of these useful devices to collect medical data may be covered by your insurance.

Step 3: Medical Summary Sheet

I prepare a summary ahead of each office visit including relevant history and questions for the doctor. This sheet accomplishes several things:

- It focuses the conversation on the issue(s) I want to discuss
- It demonstrates my baseline knowledge about the issue(s)

- It ensures that my questions will be addressed
- It ensures that, even if I bring someone along to my appointment, the conversation will be between me and the healthcare provider.

And if a doctor is under time pressure, the Summary Sheet supports an efficient use of available time.

Here is a worksheet you can complete with information about your healthcare issue. The bullet points are suggestions—you may want to make different points or ask different questions.

Summary Sheet
(Your Name) Medical Appointment for (Date)
* Potentially Relevant History
* Medication allergies or hypersensitivities
* Preexisting conditions that may be relevant
* When the current medical issue began and how symptoms have changed over time
* Any medications or other treatments so far
* Steps you are currently taking to manage the condition

Questions
* Question about causes of the condition
* Question about current medication dosages to treat the condition
* Question about other possible medications
* Question about other treatment options and next steps
* Question about prognosis

Print two copies of your Summary Sheet. When you go to your appointment, bring a clipboard with both copies of your sheet and a pen. Give one copy to the physician and hang onto the other (If there are two doctors in the room, they can share). Take notes on your copy.

If the doctor talks down, continue with your questions. If the doctor says this issue is to be expected at your age, say "I'd like to review my history and treatment options." If the doctor leaves the room without finishing the review of your history and addressing your questions, follow them down the hall and keep asking.

On the other hand, you may have the experience I had at a recent appointment: Your physician may thank you for being so "health aware" and ask if they can keep their copy of the Summary Sheet to simplify documenting the visit.

There's no need to start from scratch each time you see the doctor. Save your summary sheet on your computer and revise it for your next appointment.

Looking Ahead

This method works well when you are able to advocate for yourself. At some point we may develop medical conditions where self-advocacy is not possible. So please consider this additional step: Explain this method to whoever you have designated to advocate for you in a medical setting in the event of your incapacity, and ask them to use this approach as well.

Although the practice of medicine is conducted by fallible human beings, we can facilitate a team approach to problem solving by educating ourselves, collecting data, and providing a succinct summary of relevant history and questions. This method supports a team approach, where physicians and patients work together to address medical issues.

Becoming an active member of your care team may be uncomfortable at first, because we place our health in the hands of medical providers and want to believe they are without bias. Yet healthcare workers are human beings with human foibles, just like everyone else. Some have done the work to counter their internal ageism while others, regrettably, have not. Please advocate for yourself to receive the high level of care you deserve.

While there may be times when a physician downplays your concerns, you may also encounter the opposite problem: overprescription of medications. More about overprescription, and the deprescribing movement, in the next chapter.

And One Last Thing...

Beyond the need to manage the care we receive from healthcare providers, the care we provide to ourselves is essential. A good night's sleep and daily movement (both cardio and weight-bearing) will keep us at our best. Find ways to move that you enjoy, whether that's water aerobics, Zumba or nature walks. Check your local YMCA or other community resources.

CHAPTER 17
DRUGS AFTER SIXTY - NOT THE FUN KIND

After a career writing submissions to FDA, I was not surprised to learn that the American Geriatric Society developed the Beer's List of FDA-approved medications they recommend adults over 65 avoid. If you have ever read the package insert for a medication, you know that drug labeling lists warnings including who should not take the drug. So, you might wonder: *Why do we need the Beer's List? Doesn't FDA make drug companies study the effects of new products on older people?*

Not always. Let me tell you a story. Years ago I consulted for an organization that develops immune-based cancer therapies. My job was to write protocols for their clinical studies. In the middle of writing a protocol, I found out FDA had just published a new guidance calling for inclusion of patients over 65 in cancer clinical trials. FDA pointed out the preponderance of patients needing those drugs were in that older age group. Sounds reasonable, but think about what that means: Until that 2021 guidance, *researchers were free to exclude older people from cancer drug trials.* And what about trials for other drugs? I'd worked for decades on studies that excluded older people and never gave it a thought, until that moment in my sixties when I read the new guidance (Chalk that one up to my internal ageism).

A 2010 study pointed out that "Older adults are vastly underrepresented in clinical trials in spite of disproportionate consumption of prescription drugs and therapies, restricting treatments' efficacy and safety." (Herrera, et al.) But older adults are not the only ones underrepresented. Historically, the young white male was considered the "norm" for clinical studies. Until 1996, FDA did not require women in clinical trials. In fact, from 1977 to 1993 FDA banned women of childbearing potential from participation in early stage clinicals. People of color were often excluded from trials until passage of the Civil Rights Act in 1964 when the NIH warned drug companies that discrimination was illegal. Yet to this day, people of color remain underrepresented in clinical trials.

Patient variety in clinical trials is still an issue. In early 2025, the guidance document that required including older people and other subpopulations in clinical trials was removed by the administration (the title included the word "diversity"). And when FDA adds requirements for approval, *products already on the market do not need to meet those requirements.* As a result, data from adverse events is the only way to track whether a medication is safe and effective for a subgroup such as older people. Hence the need for the Beer's List, which includes products that treat allergies, infections, atrial fibrillation, high blood pressure, and more.

But while that list is a good idea, it is not the only word on any given medication. For example, the 2023 Beers List recommends taking women over 65 off estrogen, whereas the 2022 report by The Menopause Society says this: "There is no general rule for stopping systemic hormone therapy in a woman aged 65 years. The Beers criteria from the American Geriatrics Society has warnings against the use of hormone therapy in women aged older than 65 years. However, the recommendation to routinely discontinue systemic hormone therapy in women aged 65 years and older is neither cited or supported by evidence."

Bottom line: It pays to be a skeptical consumer of medical advice. If you are prescribed a medication on the Beers List, proceed with caution. And if you are prescribed a medication that is *not* on the list, it still pays to check the package insert that comes with the drug. A conversation with your doctor is a great next step.

Here is a case in point: Ototoxicity, or hearing loss caused by medications.

Ear Damage from Medications

Certain medications are known to risk ear damage, which can manifest as ringing in the ears (tinnitus) or as hearing loss. These hearing problems are more common among older adults. Yet ototoxicity is not cited on the Beers List. The Mayo Clinic has published a list of ototoxic medications (including a number that are not on the Beers List). So it is useful to keep both lists on hand. And keep in mind that the Mayo Clinic list is not exhaustive either. Check with your physician if tinnitus occurs when starting any new medication.

Deprescribing for Older Adults

Managing our health after sixty may involve both the dosage of medications we take and eliminating medications that cause reactions when taken together.

- **Medication Dosage:** Clinical trials study the safety and effectiveness of drugs, including the lowest dosage at which a medication does its job. The tricky part is, optimal dosage can be different for various subgroups including children, women, and older people. As we age, our ability to metabolize medications changes. A drug can stay in our system longer, meaning that a safe dose for a younger adult can be toxic for us. So unless clinical studies include older people and analyze our data as a separate subgroup, the dosage recommended on the label may be too high.
- **Multiple Medications:** While FDA requires companies to study the combined effects (cross reactivity) of certain combinations of drugs, the agency typically requires the new medication be studied with only a few drugs that are often co-prescribed. These are typically one-on-one studies: New drug A with existing drug B, and a separate study of new drug A with existing drug C. There is may be no study of A plus B plus C. Yet more than half of people over 65 report taking four or more prescription medications. For many of us, the medications we take were never studied together.

This combination of high dosage and multiple medications leads to *polypharmacy*, which is overprescription of medications to older adults. Side effects from one medication may be treated with another medication, leading to a medication cascade. The deprescribing movement recommends reviewing each individual's full range of prescriptions to carefully lower dosages and to eliminate certain prescriptions where possible. A group of Canadian researchers founded the deprescribing.org site to gather research and guidelines for this important work. For those taking multiple prescriptions, potential interactions are worth discussing with a pharmacist or primary care physician.

How to Report an Adverse Event

A woman over 65 told me she was recovering from a serious adverse reaction to a prescription drug. She notified her doctor and stopped taking the medication, but she wanted to do more. She was concerned that others might experience similar reactions. Her concern was well founded: According to a 2025 study by the American Society of Pharmacovigilance, medication reactions are the third most common cause of death in the United States. While women over 65 may be more likely to experience an adverse event, the good news is we can help protect each other by alerting FDA.

Reporting to FDA is the best way for the agency to learn about safety problems with an approved drug. If you or someone you care about has an adverse reaction to a medication, here are three ways to escalate your concerns.

- **File a MedWatch report**: Anyone who takes a medication and experiences an adverse reaction can report it directly to FDA by filing a MedWatch report online. You can report everything from a skin rash to more serious problems.

- **Ask Your Doctor to File a MedWatch Report:** FDA welcomes doctors' reports of adverse events. They even have a form designed for reports by healthcare professionals. When you talk with your doctor about your adverse reaction, you can encourage them to make a report via the physician reporting page on the FDA website. Medical journals point out that physicians have an ethical obligation to recognize and report adverse drug events.

- **Report Your Adverse Event to the Drug Manufacturer:** Look for information about filing a medication complaint on the website of the company that produced your medicine. If your reaction is significant, the manufacturer is required to make a report to FDA within days of receiving your complaint. All adverse reactions reported to the manufacturer must be logged and made available on the next inspection by the local FDA district office. The inspector will ensure that necessary corrective actions in manufacturing and testing are made.

All three of these reporting methods are important. Your MedWatch report will be reviewed by personnel at FDA headquarters in Bethesda, who look for patterns in complaints that can ultimately lead to warnings on drug labeling or even to withdrawal of an unsafe drug from the market. When you encourage your physician to submit your adverse event, their report adds weight to the seriousness of the complaint. And by filing a complaint with the manufacturer, you alert local FDA inspectors who can mandate improvements on the ground.

As FDA says on its physician reporting page, "You and your patient's report may be the critical action that prompts a modification in use or design of the product, improves the safety profile of the drug or device and leads to increased safety."

While problems with medical devices can also be reported via MedWatch, vaccines have their own reporting system. If you have an adverse reaction to a vaccine, you and your physician can report it online to the Vaccine Adverse Event Reporting System (VAERS).

When you have a health condition that requires a new medication, check to see whether the prescribed medication is on the Beers List. And if you experience an adverse reaction, do a good deed and report it. The more FDA learns about drugs that are already on the market, the better they can protect the public health.

Conclusion

It's often said, including by doctors, that the training most physicians receive in geriatric medicine barely scratches the surface. So when it comes to medications after sixty, it pays to be a savvy consumer. We have lived in our bodies for a long time and we know them well; yet our bodies change all the time, and self-care requires that we learn about ourselves as we are now. When we know more, we can partner more effectively with our healthcare providers.

CHAPTER 18
FEAR SELLS

In 2020 I signed up for a clinical study out of UCSF called the Brain Health Registry. This study of 100,000 people uses online questions and cognitive testing to gauge brain health over time. Its stated goal is to enhance research into dementia diagnosis and treatment. Each participant is asked to return every six months to revisit the questions online.

My motivation to join the study was to help fight disease. But I saw the study differently when I returned to the website in 2021 for follow-up questions. I had just finished reading Dr. Becca Levy's book, *Breaking the Age Code*. In that book, Dr. Levy summarizes her decades of research about the negative effects of internal ageism on health and longevity. Her oft-quoted statistic that people with a positive view of aging live 7.5 years longer shows that our attitudes shape our future. So the ninety minutes of questions in the Brain Health Registry, which were laser-focused on age-related decline, set off my alarm bells.

There were pages of questions about hoarding (*If emergency responders came to your home, is there so much clutter they would have trouble finding you?*). There were many questions about memory (*Do you have more difficulty remembering names than six months ago? A year ago?*). There were plenty of emotional health questions (*How often do you feel hopeless?*). There were self-care questions (*Are you able to wash your entire body by yourself?*). Totally missing were questions about developing new skills, completing new accomplishments, or sharing a lifetime of wisdom with others in our older years. Most multiple-choice questions allowed graduated responses for how badly you were doing (from slightly worse than a year ago, down to a polite version of "I suck at this"). But there was no separate answer for doing better than a year ago, just a box that combined *doing better* with *doing the same* as a year ago. For almost every question, **there was no way to stipulate positive change**.

I had just published my first novel, had judged a statewide science fair for the first time, and was lifting weights four times a week. But as I answered question after negative question, I felt less pride in my accomplishments and began to doubt myself. Maybe I did have more trouble remembering names than a year ago; how would I quantify that?

Then I began to question the motivation for the study. I "followed the money" and learned that at least one biopharma company developing dementia drugs was among the study funders. Research to support the development of new dementia drugs is extremely expensive; yet the incidence of dementia is actually falling in the United States. Could it be that these companies were trying to create a market—by adding to the internal ageism of participants and thereby damaging their cognition? I contacted the Institutional Review Board (IRB) overseeing patient safety to express these concerns.

I am a participant in the Brain Health Registry study and am concerned that the study focuses on negative effects of aging to the exclusion of any positive changes (including development of new skills and accomplishments in retirement). In fact, most of the multiple choice response options do not distinguish between doing as well as a year ago and doing better than a year ago. This is distinct from the multiple gradations for measuring decline in the responses. I recommend IRB members review the findings of Becca Levy at the Yale School of Public Health whose new book, "Breaking the Age Code," documents the negative effects on health and lifespan of the kinds of negative beliefs about aging that a study with such a negative focus might foster. While the IRB may have approved this study in the belief that it would not impact participants, Levy's studies suggest otherwise.

Three months later I received notice that the IRB had met and determined "no changes to the research surveys [were] required" to protect participants. Yet I wondered how participation in this study would affect participants who were unaware of the need to develop a positive view of aging. In 2023 I revisited the study to complete an update. There were the same old questions in a format I've come to think of as "When did you start losing your mind?" But rather than causing me to question my competence, this time I was simply annoyed by the barrage of negativity. And this time I was struck by the *product placement* in the study.

The term "product placement" typically refers to inserting a brand name into a mass media product. For example, Heineken paid $45 million for James Bond to take a sip of their beer in *Skyfall*. In this case, the dementia-related products mentioned in the Brain Health Registry survey access a valuable market of 100,000 clinical trial participants who are likely concerned about brain function.

Multiple cognitive diagnostic tests are incorporated into the study, and the companies that produce them are called out by name and thanked, right in the clinical survey. And the study now asks participants to disclose whether or not they are taking any of five different dementia medications:

- **Donepezil (Aricept)** – A medication approved in the US in 1996 that has been shown to have a small benefit for some patients in slowing Alzheimer's dementia. Common side effects include diarrhea, insomnia, and nausea.
- **Rivastigmine (Exelon)** – Used to treat mild to moderate Alzheimer's. Side effects include diarrhea and vomiting, and less commonly, aggression and convulsions.
- **Memantine (Namenda)** – Approved in the US in 2003 to treat moderate to severe Alzheimer's. Side effects include blood clots, psychosis, and heart failure.
- **Galantamine (Razadyne)** – Approved in the US to treat mild to moderate memory impairments. This medication is derived from the snowdrop and its effects were known to the ancient Greeks. Side effects include nausea and vomiting.
- **Aducanumab (Aduhelm)** – Approved in 2021 by the FDA, this expensive medication is controversial because of its high cost and serious adverse events. While the cost is reportedly $56,000 per year, forty-one percent of patients in key clinical trials experienced brain bleeding or swelling. In addition, three members of the FDA Advisory Committee quit due to safety concerns and lack of evidence of efficacy. Biogen, the manufacturer, is one of the funders of the Brain Health Registry through an intermediate organization.

Which begs the question: *How to sell products that are expensive, not very effective, and pose potentially serious risks?*

People often say that sex sells. A beautiful woman draped across the hood of a car is the stereotypical way to sell automobiles. But it's also true that fear sells. Mouthwash is sold on the fear of bad breath. Masks were sold during the pandemic on the (very real) fear of COVID. The first time I completed the questions for the Brain Health Registry, I was most concerned with its potential for direct harm to participants' cognition. This time around I saw the study as a fear-based marketing tool. The goal of the Registry may not be to damage people's health to create a market (although harm may result from repeated exposure to such slanted questions). The goal, I now suspect, is to encourage olders to focus on whatever is negative in their lives to scare them into asking their doctors for dementia medications, whether they need them or not.

Lose your keys at twenty and you're simply annoyed. Lose your keys at seventy and, *if you've been conditioned to expect dementia*, you may decide that you need medication—even expensive medication with uncertain effectiveness and potentially serious side effects. It is telling that the lead investigator's biography says he "focuses on… detecting Alzheimer's disease early in patients who are not demented, but risk subsequent development of dementia." That is to say, detecting a disease in people who don't actually have the disease.

Is marketing by fear a less sinister motivation than directly impeding cognition? Sure. But is it a legitimate reason for a 100,000-person clinical study? Not in my book.

In 2022 *Science Magazine* investigated claims that some published research papers on Alzheimer's, as well as data from a company conducting clinical trials for a dementia drug, were fraudulent. Independent reviewers found evidence that images had been tampered with in "shockingly blatant" ways, that may have misdirected Alzheimer's research for decades. The accepted cause of Alzheimer's, amyloid plaques in the brain, may be totally wrong. Yet the hypothesis that these plaques cause Alzheimer's was the standard when all of the drugs listed in the Brain Health Registry clinical survey were approved.

My outreach to the Institutional Review Board had no impact at all. But as I discussed with Margo Arrowsmith on her "Age Out Loud" podcast, if many of us enrolled in the study and contacted the UCSF IRB to express concerns, who knows? The Institutional Review Board might take a closer look. As they say at the Old School Anti-Ageism Clearinghouse, when it comes to fighting ageism, you can't start too late, and you can't start too small.

CHAPTER 19
THE LOWDOWN ON HORMONE THERAPY

Remember that long-ago day when your mother or aunt sat you down for "The Talk" about puberty? When you learned the basics about menstruation, plus (if you were lucky) a few words about sex?

Now remember the more recent day when your doctor or an older friend sat you down for "The Talk" about menopause. No? No surprise. For most of us that talk never came. And because our gonads don't come with an owner's manual, many women launch into the next phase of life not knowing much about the changes taking place and how to take care of ourselves.

In my late fifties I went to the gynecologist convinced I had a yeast infection. The burning sensation in my vulva and vagina was not responding to over-the-counter treatments. That was because I did not have an infection. Instead, I had **Genitourinary Syndrome of Menopause (GSM).** What I needed was not an anti-fungal. What I needed was topical estrogen, a cream made with estradiol, a hormone that treats the condition with minimal absorption into the rest of the body. I was incredulous. What the devil was this condition? Why didn't anybody talk about it?

The doctor gave me sample tubes of estrogen cream and said, "Be sure you don't use this as a lubricant for intercourse. Not good for your partner." When I used up the samples and had to buy it, the copay for one tube was forty dollars. Forty dollars! I was outraged. Back then I had no idea that many women who could benefit from estradiol cream were charged a lot more.

Estimates are about half of peri- to post-menopausal women have GSM. The symptoms can include burning and irritation of the vulva and vagina, dryness, discomfort with intercourse, urinary incontinence, and changes in the vaginal biome leading to recurring urinary tract infections. Nothing anybody would stand in line for. The affected structures share a common origin when we are embryos, and they are similarly affected as our estrogen levels drop with age. Tissues can thin and lose elasticity, flexibility, and blood supply.

Why GSM Often Remains Untreated

GSM can be treated with a locally applied cream made with *estradiol*, a topical hormone. Unfortunately, many women who could benefit from treatment do not receive it. This is often because they are too embarrassed to discuss their symptoms with their doctors. One study in Italy found that over 80 percent of women with GSM had not voluntarily brought up the subject with their health care providers. And, too, many doctors fail to ask enough questions to diagnose GSM. For example, asking only about discomfort during intercourse will not identify abstinent women with symptoms like urinary incontinence. As a result, about half the women in the US who could benefit do not receive treatment. And unlike hot flashes which resolve over time, the effects of GSM become more pronounced if left untreated. The upshot is that millions of women will suffer in silence, unaware of treatment or in some cases unable to afford it.

In addition, many patients and physicians in the United States are put off by the Black Box warning on the package inserts for estrogen cream. At a July 2025 FDA expert panel, available on YouTube, physicians advocated removing the warnings which are not supported by evidence.

Price has historically been another barrier. Estradiol is a steroid and a human sex hormone that is present in all genders. It has a simple chemical structure, and there is no patent on estradiol. If you buy pharmaceutical grade estradiol from a chemical supply house, you will pay $70 for a gram of pure estradiol, which is enough to make a *hundred-year supply* of estrogen cream. Yet historically the cream made from estradiol has been vastly overpriced.

One of my favorite articles on the history of drug pricing is fifty years old. "Senate Panel Cites Mark-Ups on Drugs Ranging to 7,079%" was published in the *New York Times* on December 8, 1959. Anti-trust investigators questioned Schering executives about a seven thousand percent markup on certain estrogen hormone drugs.

"Do you think this is a fair markup?" asked Senator Kefauver.

"These drugs are not an important part of our business," Schering's president replied.

"They are important to the people who need them," said the Senator.

Without insurance, and before generics were introduced, estradiol cream retailed for as much as $500 per tube. Compare that retail cost with another vaginal cream that also contains an off-patent steroid hormone: Vagisil for Sensitive Skin, a vaginal cream that contains the hormone hydrocortisone and is produced under FDA Good Manufacturing Practices, just like estradiol. The manufacturers of Vagisil are presumably making a profit at their retail price of $10 per tube.

Back in 1959, when the Senate investigated price fixing in the pharma industry, the head of Schering denied his company was charging excessively high prices for estradiol and other products. A *New York Times* article paraphrased his response: "If drug prices are high," he said, "it is because of the large costs of blazing new trails in medical research... The consumers of today must contribute to the benefits which the future will bring."

Sounds convincing, doesn't it? Certainly a whole lot better than saying "We like making gobs of money from people who need our products if they want to stay healthy." But the Senate committee didn't buy the "research" argument (and you shouldn't either). They went on to ask Schering why they were selling some products to the military for pennies on the dollar of the retail price. Pharmaceutical companies marked up estradiol by thousands of percents over manufacturing costs for fifty years, and they are selling the same product for menopausal women that they were selling half a century ago. That's a lot of "research" with no results that benefit women past menopause. Or their male partners, for that matter—half a century into the use of this product, the package insert for estradiol cream still does not say how long to wait after using the product before intercourse with a man is safe for him.

Where were the insurance companies in all this? Oral estrogen pills for contraception are priced lower and qualify for a lower deductible under many plans. But estradiol cream is seen as a drug to treat sexual health, and is typically classified as a higher tier, with the insurance company covering relatively little of the inflated cost. This means that the supplemental insurance we pay for on top of Medicare is of little value when it comes to a medication that is needed by about half the women on Medicare. A GoodRx coupon may give you a lower price than using your insurance coverage.

The introduction of generic estradiol cream eventually led to lower prices. According to a 2024 GoodRx article, pricing with their coupons can now be as low as $24 a tube. But this history stands as a lesson in the importance of raising our voices, even about sensitive products.

Systemic Hormone Therapy

Another reason women with menopause-related symptoms may not seek treatment is fear of cancer, especially with systemic hormone therapy (HT). HT supplies estrogen to the whole body, often via a patch. In their book *Estrogen Matters*, Avrum Bluming and Carol Tavris make a convincing argument that HT is an effective treatment for many health conditions related to menopause. Over the course of decades, published studies showed that HT controls post-menopausal symptoms including sleep disturbance, aching joints and depression, in addition to GSM symptoms such as vaginal dryness and frequent urination that are also helped by local application of estradiol cream. Systemic estrogen protects bone health and helps prevent osteoporosis as well as protecting brain health.

For many years, HT was prescribed to millions of post-menopausal American women. Then along came the Women's Health Initiative (WHI), a huge study that garnered much attention from medical journals and the popular press. The data from the Women's Health Initiative showed an increased incidence of breast cancer among women taking HRT. This finding was publicized widely, leading women to go off HRT in droves and physicians to stop prescribing it. But as Bluming and Tavris point out, the WHI data also showed a greater increase in breast cancer among women who eat fish and among women who are Scandinavian airline employees—not to mention women who had an extra serving of French fries in preschool. And here is the catch: *The increase for all these factors was so low that it was statistically insignificant. There was no causative link. It was just noise in the data that did not justify huge changes in women's health care.*

Yet by 2003 the use of systemic HT plummeted. Bluming and Tavris describe the process by which this meaningless data changed the standard of care for millions of women. A subgroup of trial investigators who were convinced HT was a bad idea got together and wrote a journal article touting this increase in breast cancer as if it were meaningful. The article was accepted for publication by the *Journal of the American Medical Association*. By the time the other WHI investigators saw the manuscript and objected, that issue of *JAMA* was already published and ready for distribution. And as so often happens, later corrections to the story received much less attention than the original sensational article. The damage was done, and it affects our health care today.

In fact, newer research points in the other direction. A 2024 review of the Medicare records of ten million American women over age 65 showed a 19% lower death rate during the study period for women on HT, and a 4% lower incidence of breast cancer. And even for women who have had breast cancer, newer studies are showing a *lower* rate of recurrence for women on HT. Even for breast cancer survivors like me, HT is important to our quality of life.

Every woman's body is different, and each woman has the right to determine her own care. And as we exercise that right, informing ourselves about the risks and benefits of treatment is essential. There may be no clearer example of the need to educate ourselves and speak up than the history of hormone therapy.

More to come about our bodies in the chapters that follow.

CHAPTER 20
HEALTHCARE PROFILE
BARBARA EHRENREICH

We would all like to live longer and healthier lives; the question is how much of our lives should be devoted to this project, when we all, or at least most of us, have other, often more consequential things to do.

—Barbara Ehrenreich

Barbara Ehrenreich studied physics and chemistry at Reed College and then earned a Ph.D. in cellular immunology from Rockefeller University. She gave birth to her daughter Rosa in a public clinic in New York, where, as she told *The Globe and Mail* newspaper in 1987, "they induced my labor because it was late in the evening and the doctor wanted to go home." Outraged that women in public clinics received such treatment, Ehrenreich became a feminist. She worked in health related activism for much of the 1970s and wrote extensively about the political history of women's health.

From there she branched out into other feminist journalism. Her best known book is *Nickel and Dimed: On Not Getting By in America*. For this book, Ehrenreich went undercover as a minimum wage worker living only on her earnings at various jobs: hotel maid, Walmart clerk, waitress, housecleaner. She tells her own story, including the shock of leaving her comfortable New York lifestyle for an apartment that lacked even a lock on the front door. And more importantly, she tells the stories of women living this way not just temporarily but for a lifetime.

In 2020 when she was in her seventies Ehrenreich read a *Scientific American* article describing how the aging immune system sometimes facilitates the growth of cancer rather than trying to stop it, "which is like saying that the fire department is indeed staffed by arsonists." By then this trained scientist and sceptic of the for-profit healthcare system was also a breast cancer survivor with concerns about the aggressive treatment she had received. Ehrenreich began to question how medical decisions are made. She wrote essays on overdiagnosis, overprescription, and procedures that prolong life at the expense of quality of life. At age 78 she published her treatise on reclaiming agency over our health in later life. *Natural Causes: An Epidemic of Wellness, the Certainty of Dying, and Killing Ourselves to Live Longer* invites each of us to claim control over our health as we age. Her book quotes a physician who says everyone has something wrong with them if you look hard enough.

While she emphasized that every woman should make her own decisions, Ehrenreich decided to stop humoring her doctors in the everlasting search for more diagnoses and only to consult a doctor when she had symptoms that she herself wanted addressed. She lived to age 81.

PART FIVE
BODY

Life after sixty frees us to take better care of ourselves.

Many of us put everyone else first while we juggled career and motherhood. Even when we retire and launch our children, it can be difficult to include ourselves in the circle of care, much less give ourselves priority. Negative social messages about older women's bodies can make it even more challenging to care for ourselves. But society does not own our bodies—we do. We deserve to take care of ourselves in ways that include joyful movement and self-acceptance. We get to live in our bodies like a favorite cozy robe that is comfortable and just right. As nutritionist Deb Benfield writes, "Your body is your life partner, not your life project."

The chapters that follow celebrate ways to cherish our aging bodies.

CHAPTER 21
FROM BODY NEUTRALITY TO BODY LOVE

In our society women are expected to be thin, young, and able bodied. There is only so much we can or should do to fit that impossible standard, especially after midlife, when we do not look young and when many women are naturally heavier than in our twenties.

Changes that began in our forties continue after sixty. We gradually metabolize food differently. Our body composition changes. Our skin and hair change. Our hormone levels trend downward. The differences increase between social expectations and how our bodies look, and we may judge ourselves harshly for these natural changes.

Plus after midlife, the pressure on women to meet an impossible standard of beauty collides with invisibility—the failure of others to notice us. And yet our bodies are all the more sacred, as they have carried us all these years and are serving us so well in this moment.

Right now our lungs are capturing oxygen from the air. Our bone marrow is busy making blood cells. Our intestines digest our latest meal, while our bones and muscles hold us upright. Our senses let us know what is happening around us, including the words in this book. Much of this happens without our conscious control or even our knowledge. These gifts continue every moment we live, completely separate from negative cultural messages.

One way to push back is to cultivate *body neutrality*: an attitude that values our bodies as the gifts they are without comparing them to an artificial ideal. We can look at our own bodies as the closest of friends and choose not to waste our energy on judgement. We can appreciate everything our bodies do for us right now, whether or not they look or function exactly as we wish. That attitude frees us to focus on our real priorities after sixty.

The concept of body neutrality was developed by younger women who were so troubled by society's expectations that loving their bodies was a bridge too far. Accepting their bodies and being grateful for all they do freed these women to get on with their lives. The wisdom of these younger women has great value for those of us in older bodies, as we develop the life skill of caring less about others' opinions.

If we thank our bodies for serving us well, if we practice gratitude rather than worry over each new wrinkle, we can direct our energy to rewarding our bodies for their service. That can look like moving our bodies in ways we enjoy. Swimming, bicycling, walking, weightlifting, and dancing are some of the ways to celebrate the good gift of the bodies we have now. We can express our gratitude by eating foods mindfully, focused on the tang of an orange, the texture of a walnut.

At first, a love affair with our over-sixty bodies can feel like an arranged marriage, and that is alright. We are veterans of a long struggle with the expectations of society. We can get there one step at a time.

Nutritionist Deb Benfield runs a program called "Aging with Vitality and Body Liberation" which helps women past midlife cherish our bodies so that we may live with verve. She writes, "There is nothing more powerful than learning to trust your body and yourself." Deb also places our journey in the context of how other groups are stigmatized about appearance. Her blog and her discussion groups are valuable resources. Deb's December 2025 book is *Unapologetic Aging: How to Mend and Nourish Your Relationship with Your Body*.

We are not objects to evaluate but the stars of our own lives. We can practice body love by thanking our bodies each morning for the gift of life. We can feed our senses by singing along with music we love, by viewing and creating colorful art, and by savoring delicious foods. We can move in ways we most enjoy. And we can appreciate each human body and the dignity of each person regardless of how they look. While our bodies are great gifts, our appearance is the least interesting thing about us.

CHAPTER 22
NOW YOU SEE HER, NOW YOU DON'T

It was not the threat of cancer that made me stop dyeing my hair. I saw those studies, but that wasn't the reason. I would read articles by women proudly going gray and think, *You go for it, ladies — not my thing*. I was into that conspicuously false display of reproductive fitness we create when we dye our gray hair blonde.

But I paid attention when women wrote that their hair became healthier when they stopped coloring. I was shedding everywhere. My hair clogged the vacuum. I pulled handfuls from my brush. The day finally came when I decided better gray than bald and told my partner if he wanted a blonde it was time to trade me in. He stayed on after the blonde hair landed on the stylist's floor.

After hearing friends preach the joys of invisibility, it was startling to feel myself become part of the woodwork. To fade, quite literally, into the background. To watch the eyes of men glance across me without pause, as if I were cloaked in magic. I felt loss mixed with glee at escaping the male gaze.

I had to retrain myself to see us differently, we gray haired ladies. One day I stood in the ladies' locker room at the gym, surrounded by gray haired women talking about their dogs, and caught myself thinking, *How cute they are*. I was infantilizing these women just as society does. A glance in the mirror reminded me that I was just one more gray-haired lady. We were in bathing suits headed for the pool, where a woman half our age led us in aqua fitness, all of us running clockwise in the water and creating a great current. Then at her direction we all turned and ran against the flow. Fifty women in the pool, joined by just one gray-haired man with glasses.

The instructor knew her audience; her playlist was Beatles and Frankie Valle. It was just before Valentine's Day and she asked for requests: love songs and breakup songs. We stood in rows, singing along, lunging against the water with the gray-haired man in our midst. When somebody asked for Nancy Sinatra, fifty strong alto voices boomed across the water: "One of these days these boots are gonna walk all over you." The gray-haired man startled like a rabbit, turned his head this way and that, smiled nervously. He was surrounded by a mob of women. We spend so much of our lives with that nervousness: careful where we walk at night, shining a light into the back seat before we unlock our cars, pulling the living room curtains at dusk. I indulged in a bit of schadenfreude when a man imagined himself, just for a moment, as prey.

Gray-haired women act boldly, create brilliantly, sing boisterously. Hair dye did not grant us those traits. To be our same vivid selves but not look the part is like flying under radar (For more on that, check out *Killers of a Certain Age* by Deanna Raybourn, the tale of a team of gray-haired lady assassins). But the cloak of invisibility slips sometimes when we wish it would not. Despite my gray hair, one day an older man I knew at church told me, uninvited, about his sex life, and followed me until the Ladies' Room door slammed behind me. It was eerily familiar, an echo of the ugliness of youth. I had to remind myself that I was safe and old as I set new boundaries with this overly entitled man.

A few years later I began using a tinted conditioner which leaves my hair blonde-ish, a sort of halfway place between seen and unseen. I enjoy the ambiguity.

Invisibility in our older years is a two-edged sword of freedom and loss, but visibility is a two-edged sword as well. Women want to be seen when we want to be seen. We want to walk this world strong and free, with the power to be sexual on our own terms. We should have had that power every day of our lives, but we never come close until our later years. And it is up to us to do everything we can to safeguard that agency for our daughters and granddaughters throughout their lives.

To be a sexy older woman is to claim our freedom, to live in our bodies imperfectly but as close to perfection as we will know in this lifetime.

CHAPTER 23
IF THY UTERUS OFFEND THEE

Nora Ephron had three rules for middle aged happiness: "Gather friends and feed them, laugh in the face of calamity, and cut out all the things—people, jobs, body parts—that no longer serve you."

And by body parts, Ephron meant one in particular: "The only thing a uterus is good for after a certain point is causing pain and killing you."

Amen, sister.

Have you reached that point? Has your uterus, which may once have given you that crazy impossible gift of creating an actual human being, turned on you at last? Visited upon you the entire catastrophe: endometriosis, fibroids, polyps, yearlong menstruation, and maybe even cancer?

That moment arrived for me in 2015. It's been a decade since I had my uterus (and one remaining ovary) yanked out. But that happy event was preceded by ten years of minor surgeries to pull growths that kept springing back like pink weeds. "You don't need a hysterectomy," a gynecologist assured me. "Statistics show that in our sixties, polyps stop growing back." Clearly my polyps had not seen his data. I changed doctors.

My mother had a hysterectomy because of a prolapsed uterus. Her mother had a hysterectomy because of cancer. My birth daughter is watching her back. My adopted daughter gives thanks that she's from a different lane in the gene pool.

If you've had a hysterectomy, that story may be as dear to you as birth stories are to young mothers. Giving birth to a uterus is, in a sense, the final birth story in a woman's life. And like all birth stories, it is a heroine's journey.

First comes the fight to get a doctor to agree to the surgery. This stage has the valiant quality of all insurance-driven battles, where one woman faces down an entire bureaucracy. In my case the *coup de grace* came when I happened to tell my gynecologist that my identical twin sons had been misdiagnosed as a single baby and induced two months early, and how as a result one almost died and the other rides a wheelchair. Turned out this doctor was an identical twin. She suddenly saw me as human. "When should we schedule your surgery?" was the next thing she said.

Then there is the surgery itself. Mine was an epic journey that involved untwisting a hidden ovarian tumor from neighboring organs. And then there's the recovery, when you keep feeling like you should be better by now, then overdoing it and going back to bed.

In *Spoon River Anthology*, a favorite poetry collection from a century ago, a woman kills herself after a hysterectomy. "Only the shadow of a woman after the surgeon's knife," she says. A sad tale, and you might think it outmoded. But recently I've seen memes about abortion rights that say, "If you don't have a uterus, shut the eff up." No doubt these words are aimed at men, but there are plenty of women who no longer have a uterus and have no intention of shutting up. To the women who post these memes I want to say, someday you may need a hysterectomy too. And the right to a hysterectomy when you need it may be just as important as the right to an abortion.

My mother, who grew up conversant with the Bible, was for many years a delivery room nurse. So when a gynecologist paraphrased "If thine eye offend thee, pluck it out," to replace "eye" with Nora Ephron's least favorite body part, Mom got the joke. It's hard to imagine now, but back in the 1960s gynecologists were eager for women to have hysterectomies. Mom had her surgery one brisk December morning and went Christmas shopping on the way home. That was her hysterectomy story. What is yours?

CHAPTER 24
TO BE FIT, OLD, AND FAT

My friend Nancy is in her eighties and obsessed with her weight. A small woman, Nancy is intent on becoming even smaller. She meets with a nutritionist and restricts her calorie intake, believing this will improve her health and prolong her life. At lunch she judges her own food choices, and what others are eating, out loud. Although she is ambulatory, Nancy moves very little. The idea of lifting weights to strengthen bones and muscles is foreign to her. Yet the research shows that growing stronger, not smaller, is the best thing we can do for our health as we age.

Like ageism, weight bias is a pervasive part of our culture that many accept without question. In their 2022 study, *Moving Toward Antibigotry*, the Center for Antiracist Research at Boston University identified ageism and anti-fat bigotry as the two forms of bias with the lowest recognition in the United States. Thus it can seem perfectly natural to judge ourselves and others harshly based on age or body size.

Many of us were able to fit unreasonable standards when we were young, but our weight tends to increase as we age and our metabolism slows. According to cardiologist Carl Lavie in his book *The Obesity Paradox*, the increase in fat after midlife can actually protect our health. A higher body weight is associated with better outcomes for a number of health conditions that become more likely in older age, including cancer, arthritis and diabetes.

A natural progression in weight gain after midlife can be associated with protection from falls and from succumbing to disease as the weight trend reverses. In robust people, the switch from weight gain to weight loss often occurs in the mid-sixties. Weight loss in older people can be associated with *sarcopenia*, a condition in which muscle tissue (not body fat) is lost. Emphasizing building muscle mass can be a healthier choice than trying to lose weight.

Despite a lifetime of thin propaganda, studies have shown that for women, acceptance of our weight and appreciation of our bodies increases with age. Studies also show that body acceptance is higher for people who are exposed to less advertising. The role of advertising in body shame is no surprise. There is a lot of money to be made from creating dissatisfaction with our bodies. In her book *The Diet-Free Revolution*, Dr. Alexis Conason documents that diets do not work and diet cycling can be harmful. The diet industry is built on blaming customers for its own failures. For women past midlife, many of whom are larger than the cultural ideal, weightism, ageism and sexism intersect. Self-compassion is the primary antidote for the shame that industry preys upon.

Katherine Flegal was a senior scientist at the CDC in the early 2000s when she and her team conducted a study to estimate deaths associated with weight categories defined using body mass index [BMI].

Flegal's team found that fewer than 5% of deaths were associated with "obesity" (as opposed to the 15% claimed in an earlier CDC study). The Flegal study found that "underweight" was also associated with excess deaths. On the other hand, Flegal's study found a slightly *lower* rate of deaths associated with the "overweight" category. Picture a U-shaped curve with mortality at its lowest in the middle for "overweight" individuals and higher to the left (both "underweight" and "normal" weight) and to the right (for "obese"). The CDC evaluated the Flegal study versus the earlier study and determined that Flegal's findings were a better estimate. Yet Flegal faced years of inaccurate and hostile claims about her study and her career.

Fast forward to 2014, when cardiologist Carl Lavie published *The Obesity Paradox*, a book that documents the protective effects of overweight for older persons. Dr. Lavie is one of many researchers who have found that "overweight" after sixty is associated with a lower risk of kidney failure, stroke, coronary artery disease, and other conditions. In addition, Dr. Lavie's book documents that "overweight" persons live longer and fare better than "normal" weight persons after being diagnosed with conditions including heart failure, cancer, kidney disease, arthritis and AIDS.

Given prevailing assumptions about fat and health, it is not surprising that these findings were called paradoxical. But Dr. Flegal takes issue with that term because labeling certain data paradoxical stigmatizes the data and enshrines bias. The scientific method requires researchers to base findings on data, not to judge data based on bias. Indeed, considering the U-shaped curve of mortality data, why call the weight segment associated with the lowest mortality "overweight?"

Science and medicine are conducted by human beings with inherent biases. To advocate an unbiased look at weight and health, including weight as we age, is an uphill battle. As with Dr. Flegal's findings, the "obesity paradox" has been subject to intense negative pushback from other researchers. Carl Lavie wrote: "I suddenly found myself swimming upstream against a tidal wave of ingrained ideology." In addition to scientific bias, there are financial incentives from the diet industry. A literature review in the journal *Nature* found that 67% of articles on weight loss were funded by the diet industry, and that those articles claimed much higher success rates than articles funded by non-industry sources.

More problems emerge when research translates into clinical practice. When physicians use Body Mass Index (BMI) as a basis for recommending weight loss, they employ a metric that has been called "lying by scientific authority." BMI, which is a person's weight divided by the square of their height, was developed by Adolphe Quetelet, a nineteenth century mathematician, to study population trends. Quetelet warned that BMI should not be used to estimate fat in an individual. And with good reason: BMI makes no allowance for body composition. As Dr. Lavie writes: "Bone is denser than muscle and twice as dense as fat, so a person with strong bones, good muscle tone, and low fat will have a high BMI."

It turns out that BMI is even more problematical when applied to older persons. One reason is that humans lose height over time as the discs between the spinal vertebrae flatten. This loss of height, roughly half an inch per decade after age 40, distorts the calculation of BMI. Muscle loss in older adults (sarcopenia) makes reliance on BMI even less useful—or even detrimental. An older person who loses weight because of muscle atrophy becomes less healthy, not healthier. Researchers have found that the "ideal BMI" (if there is such a thing for a metric never intended for individual use) increases as we age.

The weight loss industry targets older adults with marketing for GLP-1 weight loss drugs such as Ozempic. Clinical trials for these drugs typically enrolled 40 and 50 year olds, but the limited trial data for older adults shows a higher incidence of adverse events such as nausea, fatigue and low blood pressure. Beyond those immediate risks, rapid weight loss from these drugs can accelerate osteoporosis and muscle loss among older people, leading to frailty.

Tufts University researchers recommend that older people focus on strength training as opposed to weight loss. In addition to aerobic exercise such as walking, resistance training including hand weights and ankle weights can preserve muscle mass. Tufts University, in association with the CDC, developed a book called *Growing Stronger*, a resource that is free to download. And in 2025, researchers at the University of Virginia found "those classified as fit, regardless of BMI status, showed no statistically significant increase in CVD [cardiovascular disease] or all-cause mortality risk compared with normal weight-fit individuals."

It is not easy to question a lifetime of social conditioning about age or body size. Yet questioning these negative attitudes is essential. Dr. Becca Levy at the Yale School of Public Health found that older people with positive attitudes about aging live an average of 7.5 years longer. While I have not found a similar study about fat people who accept their body size, it seems logical that those with positive attitudes about their size would avoid extreme diets and weight cycling that are known to decrease lifespan.

Once we question those social assumptions, what can we do to construct a better path forward for ourselves?

- First, learn what the data says about our bodies as we age. Dr. Lavie's book is a great place to start. It is packed with information and research about increasing our healthspan.
- Second, move our bodies with resistance to preserve our muscles and bones. Weight training strengthens bone and prevents osteoporosis at the same time that it preserves muscle mass and prevents sarcopenia. Download the free Tufts University book to get started.
- Third, focus on body neutrality as we age. Body neutrality is the practice of appreciating our bodies for what they do for us, and recognizing that it is natural for our bodies to change over time. Acceptance and gratitude are two keys to joyful living after sixty.
- And fourth, be aware that health care practitioners may exhibit both age-based and weight-based bias. The more we know, the more we can separate fact from bias, and the more prepared we are to work with health care practitioners to protect our health as older adults.

What can we do that goes beyond each of us as individuals? My friend Nancy comes to mind: an intelligent woman who has swum in the anti-fat soup all her life and as an older woman is focused on weight loss, not strength training. I suspect that many of us know someone like Nancy. I plan to bring my friend a copy of Dr. Lavie's book and to let her know I'm open to discussing it. Will it make a difference for Nancy? I'm not sure. But if many of us take small steps, change can happen.

We are stronger when we cross barriers and see our shared struggles. For example, when disability rights advocates make common cause with the anti-ageism movement, both are stronger together. I see that same potential for common cause between the fat acceptance movement and the anti-ageism movement. Ultimately, all forms of bigotry are anti-humanist. When we push back on prejudice of every kind, we free ourselves to live our best lives.

Appreciating and taking care of our bodies can include mindful eating and regular body movement along with size acceptance. To focus on behaviors rather than body size helps us love and accept our bodies. Enjoying what we eat is part of our birthright as humans. Our later years can be a time to appreciate the sweet fruits of Planet Earth.

By loving our bodies in all these ways—by expanding our concept of beauty, by movement, by the enjoyment of food—we prepare ourselves for what can be our best, most rewarding years. We can expand the range of who we see as beautiful to include ourselves—the subject of the next part of this book.

CHAPTER 25
BODY PROFILE
DR. KATHERINE FLEGAL

According to some of our critics, new and better scientific results are dangerous and cause confusion if they fail to buttress what you already believe.

—Dr. Katherine Flegal

During a thirty-year career as a researcher at the Centers for Disease Control (CDC), Dr. Katherine Flegal published articles showing that American's average weight was increasing. These articles were readily accepted by academic obesity researchers. Her strong background in nutrition and statistics was well known, and her careful analysis of data was widely acknowledged.

Then in 2005 Flegal and her team published a thoroughly researched article in the *Journal of the American Medical Association* showing that people classified as "overweight" lived longer on average than those

135

considered "normal" weight, and people classified as "obese" had lower mortality than previously thought.

Although the article was based on the same kinds of careful data analysis, the response from academics was an aggressive campaign of rumors, misinformation, and phone calls to her superiors. Within hours of publication in *JAMA*, Dr. Flegal was fielding calls from journalists who had already been contacted by a faculty member at Harvard complaining about her findings. An entire symposium was organized at the Harvard School of Public Health to dispute her findings. The well-documented results were described in unprofessional terms such as "rubbish," "ludicrous," "complete nonsense." Baseless attacks in presentations at scientific conferences, as well as in published literature, continued for years. For example, a post doctoral fellow at Harvard published an article stating that Flegal had been demoted at CDC as a result of the study (in fact, Flegal's *JAMA* article earned her the Shepherd Award, CDC's highest honor for scholarly work). Dr. Flegal has expressed concern that this type of behavior may intimidate other researchers whose findings do not conform to the accepted paradigm about body size. She herself was undeterred. Flegal believes that science should be based on data, not on whether it fits a commonly held narrative.

After she retired from the CDC, Flegal became a professor at the Stanford University School of Medicine. Former FDA Commissioner David Kessler called her "one of the great epidemiologists." Her article, *"The Obesity Wars and the Education of a Researcher,"* is Flegal's personal account of the manufactured controversy about her research.

∼

PART SIX
BEAUTY

We are taught to associate beauty with youth, to see beauty through the lens of fertility. What if we took off those blinders and viewed one another from a different vantage point: not ignoring the beauty of the smooth-skinned young, but expanding our range to include the loveliness of the Mother, the comeliness of the Queenager, the elegance of the Crone. What would we see?

And what if we focused as well on beauty of character and the beauty of hard-earned wisdom?

These chapters on Beauty explore this wider vision.

CHAPTER 26
LET SHE WHO GROWS HER CHIN HAIRS CAST THE FIRST STONE

Prejudice is not about how we look. It's about what people in power want our appearance to mean.
—Ashton Applewhite

I have had it up to here with women who critique other women's appearance—and that includes me. I was totally judgmental back in 2023 when I saw the photos of Madonna at the Grammys. Her look after plastic surgery provoked an uncanny valley reaction: Madonna looked to me like an android, like an attempt to make a human face from clay. And then I read what Madonna thought about reactions like mine, because she had been subjected over and over to misogyny and ageism. I had aligned myself with the problem even though I know damned well that when women find it necessary to change our bodies to meet career expectations, the issue is about the system, not the woman.

By the time Martha Stewart's *Sports Illustrated* cover came along, I knew to expect the attacks, many from other women: *Martha at 81 must have had some "work" done to look that good; Martha was photoshopped.* And of course, the old standby: *Martha can't possibly be a natural blonde at that age.*

Step back a minute and think how many magazine covers feature younger women who have had plastic surgery; younger women who are photoshopped; younger women who dye their hair. Now ask yourself: *Why is an older woman supposed to be purer than Caesar's wife, while younger models get a pass?*

The magazine was criticized, too, for choosing this particularly privileged older woman. But let's put that choice in context. For years, *Sports Illustrated* swimsuit covers were an endless parade of thin young blonde white women. More recently women of color have been featured, and in 2021 a trans woman appeared on the swimsuit cover. The magazine still has a way to go; I would love to see Lizzo on the cover. But the choice of an 81-year-old woman—regardless of privilege—is a first step away from age bias.

Sniping about the appearance choices of women after midlife is not only counterproductive, it also betrays, as Madonna pointed out, a whole lot of gendered ageism. And on top of that, when older women critique each other about our looks, we reveal a surprising level of bias—even among women in the anti-ageist community. Purity testing about appearance can also have a religious aspect. Believe it or not, there are websites where fundamentalist women talk about "God-Given Gray." The premise is that when a woman's hair turns gray, God did that, so we should leave it alone. I want to ask these women: *But didn't God also make hairs sprout on your chin after menopause? Do you grow out your chin hairs as a sign of purity?*

With that in mind, I've come up with a new standard: *Let she who grows her chin hairs cast the first stone.* In other words, before a woman critiques another for failing some kind of test about her "natural" appearance, the critic should make sure that she herself is absolutely pure.

Ladies, here are some criteria for your personal purity test:

- **Do you grow your chin hairs?** No? Then stop criticizing women who also modify their appearance.
- **Have you stopped wearing brassieres** out of concern they might oppose the effects of gravity on your aging body? No? Ditto.
- **Have you thrown out all your makeup** because even lipstick might disguise your age? No? Ditto again.
- **Have you given up trying on clothes** before you buy them, for fear that your choices might be flattering? No? Bingo.

Bottom line: Unless you're on the pure side of each criterion, please back off.

It would be sexist to expect more from older women than from older men. And given that men are generally less bothered by chin hairs, they need a different purity test before they criticize older women's appearance.

So, men, let's try out this test:

- **Have you stopped wearing deodorant?** No? Then you're not pure enough to criticize how Women of a Certain Age present ourselves to the world.

- **Do you still wear T shirts from your teen years even if they don't fit?** No? Ditto.
- **Did you buy your first sportscar after age 50?** Come on. Don't even open your mouth.
- **Are you, in fact, a woman?** No? Then give it up.

How about it, guys? Did you pass all four? (And I didn't even ask about the Little Blue Pill; I'm taking it easy on you fellas.)

Everyone of every gender faces age discrimination. But we know from the research that ageism and appearance discrimination affect women earlier and more significantly than men. So let's stop the criticism of older women for adaptations of every type, from ditching our chin hairs all the way to Botox. If we want to criticize something, let's focus on the systemic issues that push women to make these choices.

And, too, let's celebrate the freedom we have as older women to express ourselves, through our actions as well as appearance. Let's cheer Women of a Certain Age who wear "inappropriate" clothing and date younger men. Let's applaud older women who lift weights, write novels, and start companies. Women who resume the passions of our youth, or find new passions after fifty, sixty, and beyond: Making jewelry, growing roses, charting the stars.

Strong women become stronger by lifting each other up. Let us do what we love and support other women in their choices.

CHAPTER 27
TOWARD A NEW DEFINITION OF BEAUTY

The anthropologist Margaret Mead married a series of men, each one a researcher about to travel to a place she wanted to study. At the end of an assignment she divorced and married anew. An extreme method, perhaps, and yet it enabled Mead to examine and write about cultures all over the planet. Decades later, when her work was famous throughout the first world, it amused Mead that her invisibility as an older woman enabled her to visit remote cultures on her own and ask a thousand questions almost unnoticed.

Is invisibility after menopause a superpower or a detriment? If we want to observe unhindered, invisibility can be marvelous. If we want to seduce someone, invisibility is inconvenient. The answer depends on what we want to do.

And then there are women who are strikingly noticeable long past midlife. Iris Apfel was the antithesis of the invisible older woman. Apfel, who developed an interest in fashion as a young child, became a fashion model in her eighties after a stunning career in fashion and textiles. She published her eponymous book in 2018 with the subtitle "Musings of a Geriatric Starlet." Her advice is a recipe for continuing to shine: Wear bold glasses, red lipstick, a big necklace, bracelets on both arms, and dress to please yourself. Hit the vintage stores when budget is an issue. Apfel brought joy and play to our definition of beauty with every bright outfit she wore.

The key thing is to own our visibility. Like a super-heroine with a cloak of invisibility, we can choose when to be seen and when not to be. Among the many lessons of the marvelous Ms. Apfel, who lived to 102: We can keep playing with our choices even past the century mark.

A new understanding of beauty is emerging. Joyce Tenneson's book *Wise Women* collected photographs of women ages 65 to 100, celebrating their extraordinary beauty. Connie Brisco's book *Stepping Out* celebrates, as its subtitle says, *The Unapologetic Style of African Americans Over Fifty*. Meanwhile older women models expand our view of beauty in every season. Professor Lyn Slater was 63 when she launched her fashion career as the "Accidental Icon." And centenarian Iris Apfel delighted us with her extravagant sense of style. Her mantra: Never wear one necklace when you can wear five.

Youth is not synonymous with beauty. When we view images like these, and the stunning photography in Ari Cohen's *Advanced Style* books, we begin to see beauty more broadly than we did before. We see our own beauty more clearly.

How we express our beauty is part of our agency as women. For many women, natural silver locks are a symbol of pride in this stage of life. Other women whose hair turns gray dye their hair because they enjoy how they look, or to make themselves more appealing to ageist employers. As with all life choices, to dye or not to dye is part of each woman's agency. After all, if women as a group were to stop changing our appearance to match the expectations of society, then all women—not just older women—should stop dying our hair. By the same token, we should all, young and old, stop wearing makeup. Until that day arrives, it's only right that women of every age should enjoy the same freedom of appearance.

When biologist Barbara McClintock belatedly won the Nobel Prize for her work in genetics, she reluctantly bought a new dress and bemoaned women's "cultural obligation to be decorative." McClintock reminded us that even beyond expanding the definition of beauty, we can honor the inherent worth of all people, regardless of appearance.

CHAPTER 28
THE LEGS ARE THE LAST TO GO

One hot summer day I was walking into the grocery store in shorts when a young man ahead of me glanced over his shoulder and gave me the once-over. He started at my feet and looked interested, then quizzical, then somewhat abashed as his gaze travelled from conventionally attractive legs to my round middle to my sixty-something face. At that point he turned and scurried through the door.

That incident reminded me of another woman's guilty post. She asked how she could consider herself anti-ageist when she loves being told she looks young for her age. Exactly. I want to have it both ways: I want to be revered for my wisdom yet seen as attractive (which in our culture, so far, means young).

The actor Jamie Lee Curtis is a reformed plastic surgery client who tells her daughters, "Don't mess with your face." Going under the knife must be such a temptation in Hollywood, where a woman's last fuckable day is her fortieth birthday. It must be tough to live in a company town where one's entire standing is based on superficialities (Not that the rest of the country is all that deep).

But you never hear about a woman having plastic surgery on her legs. And why is that? Because the legs are the last to go (*"Go where?"* You might ask. *"Doesn't 'the last to go' mean 'the last to change with age?' Isn't that ageist?"* Yes—duly noted). We should start a new fashion trend: short dresses for seventy-year-olds. Let's show our pretty knees. And while we're at it, let's dye our hair any color we want, just like women half our age do all the time. Ask yourself what makes you feel sexy and alive and then go do those things.

Some of us who want to be anti-ageist take guilty pleasure in being told we look young for our age. When someone compliments us with that you-look-younger nonsense, perhaps it's best to say: "I'm glad you think I'm attractive." Not "*still* attractive," just attractive. Or, "I'm glad you see beauty in me." Because we need to unlink youth from beauty. And we need to unlink beauty from worth.

Photographer Jocelyn Lee photographed naked older women for 35 years to create her 2020 monograph, *Sovereign*. She writes eloquently about why she developed this project:

The unclothed body is our primary vessel, sensual home, and gateway to the rest of the world. As women age into their fifties, they become not only invisible, but experience a denial of their bodies as a locus of sensual pleasure. The idea of an older woman feeling sexy, happy, and comfortable in her naked body is often met with disgust and discomfort.

And yet that is how we are, or can be: sexy, happy and comfortable in our naked bodies, loving them like we love our favorite sweater. The defining scene in the marvelous movie *Good Luck to You, Leo Grande*, is the moment when Emma Thompson gazes at her naked self in the mirror, standing in that Eve-in-the-Garden stance, one leg slightly bent. She is transformed by pleasure, looking on her body with gratitude and joy. She has come home to her body at last. Remember that saying: "The Revolution will not be televised?" In that moment, revolution came to the screen. Thompson invited each of us to a moment with the mirror. She called us to a different way to see our bodies. Love begins with self-love, and the appreciation of our beauty begins with us.

What we are seeing now in books, movies, and television shows is the upswelling of a new culture. It is a culture that opposes gendered ageism, a pro-aging culture that embraces the beauty and wisdom of older women. As Jocelyn Lee wrote, "It's time we revolutionize the image world and flood it with women in real bodies, feeling sensual and wonderful in their human skin."

What begins with each of us will expand to all of us. Let's look at one another with appreciation for our beauty, regardless of our age, gender, body type, race, or abilities. And let's see beyond beauty, to the inherent worth in each of us.

My wish for that young man at the grocery store is that he will grow in wisdom and come to see each woman as another human soul on the same mortal journey.

CHAPTER 29
THE TALE OF THE PEACOCK

What have tail feathers ever done for the peacock? They are heavy, they harbor parasites, and they add nothing to the bird's ability to eat, drink, or move. So why have they persisted generation after generation?

A peacock's tail is an example of an elaborate display of reproductive fitness. The apparent basis for the tail's attraction: A bird that has so much energy to waste on mere display must have plenty going on as a potential mate.

While the male bird is the one with the big feathers, in humans it is the female who carries the burden of decorative display. Any woman who has wedged her feet into pointed shoes knows all about appearance and courtship rituals. Studies have shown that males pay more attention to the appearance of females than women do to men's looks. And the visual cues males seek in courtship are signs of fertility, which are tied to youth. No wonder there are multibillion dollar industries that depend on the female demand to conform to youthful appearance standards: the makeup industry, the diet industry, the cosmetic surgery industry, all of them powered by evolutionary biology.

We know that human women, unlike other species, live way past our reproductive years. In evolutionary terms, it makes sense that human males would avoid mating with late-life women (or it made sense in the past; overpopulation is no concern of evolution). But in human terms, from the sexy midlife woman's point of view, it can make sense to display signs of reproductive fitness long after those signs no longer apply. As a woman who went grey at forty and tints her hair decades later, I am amazed at how much that one little signal of long blond hair changes how people react.

Blond hair on a woman is a lot like a big tail on a peacock: It is a conspicuous display that may be completely inaccurate but still conveys an advantage. When I read articles about what older women should not wear, or whether we should dye our hair, I wonder whether the writers of those articles understand the ancient game we are playing. We don't just fool each other when we stage these displays. We fool our DNA.

CHAPTER 30
BEAUTY PROFILE
LYN SLATER

Age is never a variable I use to make decisions about what I wear.

—Lyn Slater

Fashion was always a mode of creative expression for Lyn Slater, but it became her career in her sixties. Slater, now retired from a professorship at Fordham University, began her work life in a locked facility for delinquent adolescent girls. She came to see the issues there not as crime but as the result of trauma and neglect these young women experienced as girls. Slater became head of a sexual abuse project at a law firm and was frequently called to testify. She paired cowboy boots with the dark suits she wore to court for just a hint of personal style. After the law firm she earned a Ph.D. in social work and was recruited by Fordham University to found an interdisciplinary program linking the schools of law and social work.

All this time Slater developed her style and collected fashion, mostly second hand designer clothing from thrift stores. She was discovered by fashion journalists and started her Accidental Icon Instagram at age 61. Her self-confidence and distinctive style combined with her grey hair made Lyn's page a huge draw for other women who refused to be invisible. As she wrote, "A grandmother with grey hair and wrinkles became a fashion star."

At first it was great fun to work with emerging designers. But as an Instagram influencer with hundreds of thousands of followers, plus modeling contracts with major fashion houses, Slater discovered that fashion was more of a business than the creative outlet she had always enjoyed. The role of Instagram influencer turned into a 24/7 job. She spent enormous amounts of time on the telephone and communicating with followers. Eventually Lyn had to step aside and decide what to do next.

In addition to her love of fashion, Lyn had always wanted to write. When she decided to write a book, she was chagrined to realize that her agent and her publishing contract came to her because of her Instagram platform, not because of her literary chops. She wanted to be worthy of her success.

Her book, *How to Be Old: Lessons in Living Boldly from the Accidental Icon*, is a memoir of Slater's sixties and how she lived that decade as an icon. As her sixties approached, Slater was inundated with AARP invitations and cemetery plot flyers. She wrote:

How old I am is hands down the most boring fact about me. I became determined at age fifty-nine not to let age define me, or get in my way. All the reminders that I was getting old only served to provoke me. They fueled my desire to make this decade one where I will resist stereotypes that dictate what I should look like or how I should live life when I am old.

In this insightful book, Lyn Slater reinvents herself yet again.

PART SEVEN
MONEY

Most American women work two shifts: An underpaid shift in the daytime and an unpaid Second Shift caring for household and children. All too many of us emerge at the end of our careers with lower savings and lower Social Security than our male counterparts, which must sustain us for a longer lifespan. These chapters explore strategies to manage our financial power and support our freedom after sixty.

Many topics in this book (such as Creativity and Purpose) are timeless. A few (and in particular this topic of money) can change with government policies on Medicare, Social Security, and more. Please consult the blogs and conversations at www.stellafosse.com as well as your financial advisor as we navigate these changes.

CHAPTER 31
WORK SUCKS FOR WOMEN TOO

Years ago I worked with a woman who won nine million dollars in the California state lottery. The lottery folks suggested she take a monthly payout but she said no thanks, she wanted it all. After taxes her payout was just over three million dollars.

This woman – let's call her Claire – was the administrative assistant in the Marketing department. I didn't know her personally, but my friends would point her out at company picnics. "That's Claire," they would say. "She's the one who got three million dollars and *did not quit her job.*"

There's a side note to this story that I must tell you. Back before she won the lottery, Claire's old Honda was stolen one night. She reported the theft to the police but in her view, they did not do enough to track down her car. So Claire drove her rental around town until she spotted her stolen car, then called the police and told them to come get it. Which they did. After Claire became a multimillionaire, she still drove that beat up Honda to work.

Back then I was fixated on Claire. I used to fantasize what I would do if somebody handed me three million dollars. None of my fantasies involved staying at my job, although my job was arguably more interesting than being the admin for the Marketing department. I suspected that Claire suffered from a failure of imagination. I wondered if she might enjoy a complimentary brainstorming session to get in touch with her creative side. Common sense prevailed, for once, and I left her in peace.

I quit that job decades ago, but Claire still crosses my mind. In more recent years I've thought that perhaps she, like many women of my generation, was so busy proving that women could succeed in the workplace that she did not have the bandwidth to consider work more critically. Sure, there are all kinds of books and articles about how tough it is for women to balance motherhood and career (Motherhood. As if every child born was a reenactment of the Virgin Birth). But spilling the beans on the dirty little secret that work itself sucks, aside from the parenting angle, seems largely to be the province of men who don't need to prove they belong on the job.

And I have to say that some of these guys are great at trashing the hyper-work ethic. Jackson Browne in "The Pretender," singing about being a happy fool in the struggle for money, is an all-time favorite. And then there is Luo Huazhong who responded to the insanely long work hours in China by founding the "lie flat" movement. He only rises on occasion to play a few video games for a little cash. And Tim Kreider, whose *New York Times* article "It's Time to Stop Living the American Scam" proclaims, 'To young people, America seems less like a country than an inescapable web of scams, and 'hard work' less like a virtue than a propaganda slogan, inane as 'Just say no.'"

Fantastic stuff.

But I am glad to see women joining the work-bashing chorus. A former NPR reporter, Cassady Rosenblum, wrote a *New York Times* article proclaiming, "Work is a False Idol." Another young woman's tweet that she didn't want a career, she wanted to sit on the porch, has been retweeted 75 thousand times.

The United States has a worker shortage (or at least a young worker shortage) along with, apparently, a baby shortage. My response to the caterwauling about both issues: You get what you incentivize. If workers are expected to put in long hours for lower real wages than their forebears, if the social supports that exist for parents in other first world countries do not exist here, well, *what do you expect?*

Predictably, the worker shortage has spawned a rash of articles about workplace opportunities for retirees. Because older people suffer from ageism in hiring, some of us have the same urge to compensate and prove ourselves that women had back in the day. But before we jump back in, let's stop to remember why we retired in the first place. Just what is life like for workers in the United States?

In 2021 Goldman Sachs produced a report on its worker satisfaction. Now, granted, not every work environment is as high-pressure (or as highly paid) as Goldman. But just consider: On average, first year analysts were working 105 hours a week and sleeping five hours a night. One person commented they had a total of four hours a day to cook, eat, do laundry, shower, interact with friends and family, and use the bathroom. Most respondents reported they were unlikely to still be working at Goldman Sachs in three months. But that begs the question: *Just where were they planning to go?*

Women who did not win three million in the California lottery face multiple financial challenges in retirement. We spent our careers earning lower wages than men, leading to lower retirement savings and smaller Social Security payments. We are more likely to take time away from the workforce for childrearing and other caretaking, affecting our ability to save. And when we return to work, we typically take a 20% hit in earnings. Then we must make those lower savings last over a lifespan that averages five years longer. One panelist in a presentation at the Milken Institute called it the "march toward poverty." As she put it, "the math does not work." With those numbers in mind, a return to work may seem like a great idea, or the only idea.

But before we celebrate the new gray workforce, before we put on our rose-colored glasses and fondly remember the bosses we could not stand at the time, let's consider our options. Gloria Steinem famously said, "One day an army of gray-haired women may quietly take over the Earth." Perhaps we will take over by sitting quietly on the front porch, only rising on occasion to get paid to play a few video games. Let us cherish our hard-won freedom and reimagine how to keep it.

CHAPTER 32
FINANCIAL STRATEGIES AFTER SIXTY

At the start of the Industrial Revolution, labor theorists saw the transition from small business owner to factory employee as a kind of servitude. The contrast between that view and the American worship of work could not be clearer. And yet the times are changing.

Over the course of the COVID-19 pandemic, the rate of retirement doubled—a trend that was dubbed the "Great Retirement." But we older Americans were not alone; many people of working age began to deprogram from the cult of work. The "Great Resignation" was the most visible facet of a large movement to regain agency in our lives. This cultural shift happened because people of every age came face to face with mortality. Twenty percent of Americans lost someone close to them in the pandemic. Life expectancy in the United States declined for the first time in decades. Older and younger workers realized that life becomes more precious when the number of our days is up for grabs.

While many of us either wanted to retire or were forced to do so, we did not all approach this new stage in life with the same financial security. There is huge variety in the financial status of older people, especially older women. At one end of the spectrum, women of wealth are changing the nature of philanthropy, with a greater focus on programs that benefit women and girls. At the other extreme, the number of homeless older women is growing. Yet the subject of money is considered taboo. Many women with few resources are embarrassed to talk about their circumstances. Wealthy women can be reticent to speak about their status due to feelings of guilt that they have more than others.

As we age, our relationship with money inevitably changes. It is important to talk about where we stand financially, how to manage this powerful force in our lives, and the public policy changes that could make life better (or worse) for older women in the future.

Why Money is Tougher for Women

If you have left the workforce or are considering it, and unless you are wealthy, you may be up against four factors that make money tougher for older women.

- The lower pay we received throughout our careers due to gender discrimination means lower lifetime savings and lower Social Security.
- Women are more likely to take time away from the workforce to raise children or care for aging family members—again resulting in lower savings and lower Social Security.
- Workplace ageism affects women earlier than men. Women are likely to be overlooked for promotions (or pushed out

of careers altogether) at an earlier age than male colleagues.
- Women live longer than men and must make their smaller savings last longer. As a result, the demise of traditional pensions and the switch to retirement savings plans hurt women more than men.

And on top of all that, a *New York Times* study found that women's retirement savings are tapped more often when adult children need help.

Let's consider what money looks like for women at each economic stratum, and how women can improve our own status and help others.

When Money is Tight

With the days of defined benefit plans behind us, and given that women live longer on less, it is no surprise that the median savings and income of older women are lower than for men. On top of that, there is a wealth gap between older women of color and older white women. In addition to a lifetime of discrimination in hiring and wages, women of color are less likely to have had family financial support for college and for home purchases, making it more difficult to accumulate wealth. Women of color are also less likely to inherit wealth. Fortunately, there are ways for older women to improve our financial circumstances.

On the **income** side, some women are willing and able to continue fulltime work into their sixties or even seventies. Doing so increases available savings and can allow women to delay taking Social Security benefits, increasing the monthly payout. Other women will not or cannot continue to work full time. For these women, a combination of income streams can help.

- **Explore part time work and the gig economy.** Part time work may be in the field where you worked most of your life but could also be something you enjoy and have not had a chance to explore during these busy middle years. Some women set up Etsy stores to sell their crafts. Others drive an Uber part time. Consider creating a collective: a group of older women with related skills who band together to provide services. This could be anything from pet sitting to driving children to after school activities.
- **Apply to programs that help older workers** to re-enter the work force. The AARP Foundation Back to Work 50+ Program is one example, and there may be others in your local area.
- **Think about renting out extra bedrooms** if you have them. Older women can join forces to create Golden Girl households, meeting social as well as financial needs. There are now services to help women find suitable matches for these households.
- **Look at taking Social Security early** as part of your income stream. Much has been written about the advantages of waiting until full retirement age, but that assumes a long life. To take an extreme example, a woman who takes benefits at age 62 and dies at 64 clearly receives more than if she had decided to defer until 66. The Social Security Administration calculated benefits such that a person who dies on their 88th birthday receives exactly the same amount no matter when they began to collect benefits. If a woman dies after 88 she is better off waiting as long as possible to collect. If a woman dies before 88 she is better off taking lower benefits earlier. And given that we

don't know when we will die, it makes sense to factor our circumstances into the timing decision. In addition, check your earnings history on the Social Security website. Social Security is based on a worker's top 35 earning years. If you worked fewer than 35 years, your benefits calculation factors in zeroes for the missing years. This means that if you work part time after you begin collecting benefits, your benefits will be recalculated each year, and will increase after each additional year of income. Thus it can make sense to take benefits early and keep working part time. Bear in mind, though, that if you claim benefits before your full retirement age and earn more than the yearly earnings limit in a given year, your benefits will be reduced for that year by $1 for every $2 you earned. The yearly earnings limit for a given year is listed on the Social Security website, and only applies until you reach full retirement age.
- And speaking of benefits: **Learn about other benefits you qualify for, and then apply.** For example, AARP has found that most people over 65 who qualify for SNAP (formerly known as food stamps) do not take that benefit. Asking for help when we need it is an important life skill. While our society prizes the "rugged individual," the reality is that we are all interdependent throughout our lives.

Here are ideas to consider on the **expense** side of the ledger.

- **Take advantage of senior discounts**: Your local grocery store may offer a senior discount on a certain day of the week. Movie theaters may have senior matinees and some restaurants have a discounted senior menu.
- **Consider downsizing**: You may not need all the room your family required earlier in life. And while many of us want to live independently as long as possible, that

independence may last longer in a smaller, one-story home that costs less and is easier to maintain. Our health can change quickly and unexpectedly. The time to make a move and harvest our equity is while we have the strength to do it.
- **Find creative ways to lower expenses**: Split a restaurant entrée with a friend. Go to a pay-as-you-can café. Organize a group of friends to share potluck meals and trade services with one another. For example, one of those shared services can be helping one another downsize, sell possessions, and move into smaller dwellings.

Older women who are struggling financially may also find that volunteer work improves their outlook and can lead to new skills and employment opportunities.

When Money is Flush

Women who have pursued well-paid careers, did not take time off for childrearing, or inherited money from parents or husbands may be well off despite the ups and downs of the stock market. Older women in this category are changing philanthropy in the United States to emphasize organizations that benefit women and girls. High profile examples of women philanthropists include:

- Jennifer Buffett heads the NoVo Foundation, one of the largest family foundations run by a woman. It awards $55 million each year, with its primary mission to empower women and girls as agents of change worldwide.
- MacKenzie Scott gave away six billion dollars of her fortune in 2020. Scott, who founded Amazon with her former husband, is known for careful research, giving

without conditions, and wide-ranging support of such organizations as historically Black colleges, community colleges, and non-profits. She has signed the Giving Pledge, whose signatories commit to give away half their wealth in their lifetimes or through their wills.
- Melinda Gates founded the Maverick Collective in 2016 to bring together female philanthropists. When Gates signed the Giving Pledge, she wrote, "I commit my time, energy and efforts to the work of fighting poverty and advancing equality—for women and other marginalized groups—in the United States and around the world."

Other women of means band together to form giving collectives through organizations such as the Women's Funding Network. Founded in 1984, this organization connects leaders with tools and resources to empower women and girls worldwide.

This model of collective sharing, which has long been a hallmark of African American culture, is beneficial for all women, especially as we age. As Ashton Applewhite has written, "Aging is a team sport."

Women in the Middle

For many women, our savings plus our expected Social Security payments may or may not last until the end of life, depending on how long we live and how significant our care expenses will be at the end of life. Neither wealthy nor yet in poverty, we have more constraints than wealthy women but may have more options than women in reduced circumstances. Our choices include:

- **Entrepreneurship**: While we may not be in a position to stop earning money completely, we may also have the means to establish ourselves with a new venture that reflects our passions. Older entrepreneurs are often more successful because of our well-developed skills, our extensive networks, and because Medicare enables us to work for ourselves without worrying about health insurance. The first step to become an entrepreneur is to assess our skills and investigate unmet needs to determine where our strengths can best be used. For those new to entrepreneurship, cultivating curiosity, a learning mindset, and a willingness to take reasonable risks are important. In addition, becoming certified as a woman-owned business can increase sales. Certain potential customers, such as Target and Starbucks, give preference to women owned businesses as suppliers. Therefore certification through the Women's Business Enterprise National Council can provide a competitive advantage.
- **Social Security**: As stated earlier, if we have worked fewer than 35 years for reasons such as childrearing, we can increase our benefits through income later in life. Once we reach full retirement age, there is no decrease in benefits regardless of our income level.
- **Housing Options**: Downsizing, or setting up a Golden Girls household, are options that were discussed earlier. We can also consider cohousing. Cohousing is a form of cooperative housing in which each household has its own relatively small housing unit and shares common facilities, typically including a communal kitchen, meeting rooms, and guest quarters which the residents can book for visiting family and friends. There are usually twenty to forty households in a cohousing community, and many older women are involved in the cohousing movement. In cohousing, many meals and other activities are shared by the group. This type of community living promotes

interactions and friendship. Cohousing originated in Denmark and has expanded in recent decades in the United States. There are roughly 150 cohousing communities in the US, most with a mix of ages, but some are designed as senior communities where the guest quarters may eventually be converted to caretaker living quarters. More communities are in the planning stages. Whatever our housing choices, it is important to remember that accessible housing will make it easier to remain in our homes later in life. The time to make those changes is now, while we have the resources and energy to do so.

Raising Our Voices

All of us, no matter our income or assets, can support public policies that will benefit today's older women and those coming up.

- First of all, we can advocate for the kinds of financial supports that make older homelessness less likely in other countries.
- Second, we can advocate for increasing the income cutoff for contributions to Social Security. This will support the continued health of the Social Security system.
- Third, we can advocate for a guaranteed floor on Social Security payments. This is in line with the guaranteed income movement which is being tried in several parts of the country.
- Fourth, we can advocate for increased funding for home care. Most Medicare funding for adults who need support with activities of daily living goes to nursing homes, even though nursing home care is more expensive and most adults who need those supports would prefer to remain at home.

- We can advocate for expansion of the Hospital at Home movement, which enables many who require hospitalization to be transferred to their own homes and continue to receive hospital-level care.
- We can also advocate for more accessible housing, to benefit people of every age who have or acquire mobility issues.

We must recognize the under-recognized, the workers whose toil is too physically demanding, too stressful, or just too boring to continue through our sixties and beyond. The people advocating late life work are not stocking shelves at Walmart. And they may unwittingly give comfort to those who would take away the Social Security savings we paid into our whole lives.

We are More Than Our Careers

Work can be intellectually stimulating and socially rewarding. It also consumes our free time, depletes our energies for the things we are passionate about, and diminishes our connections with families and friends. Although our culture glorifies work, a recent study found that of forty life activities, only being sick in bed caused people more misery than work. And yet, in the United States, one of the first questions we ask one another when we first meet is, "What do you do?" As we transition away from the careers in which we spent so much of our adult lives, we get to redefine who we are and how we want to answer that question. What we do now is not what we did. "I was an accountant" makes no more sense than saying "I was a college student."

"I am a consultant" covers a lot of ground. "I am an Uber driver" is a fine and respectable new career. And consider the possibility of answering with your passion instead of the way you make money. When asked what you do, "I am a writer" is a perfectly good answer, well before a publication date. So is "I'm an artist." Money is powerful, but the way we make our money is not who we are.

Let's live our whole lives, not just our careers. Work need not be servitude. Whether we are, or have been, consultants or employees, our skills are valuable, but not as valuable as the people we love—including ourselves.

CHAPTER 33
MEDICARE FOR SOME

When I turned 65, it was time to choose my Medicare pathway. The choice took five minutes. I knew nothing about Original Medicare, MediGap plans, and Medicare Advantage plans (except that Original Medicare sounded a bit like KFC Original Recipe). So I chose the Medicare Advantage insurer that advertised "the only Medicare plans with the AARP name, for more than 20 years. These plans stand for quality, value and service."

That quote is from an ad in the October 2023 *AARP Bulletin*, sent to all 38 million AARP members just in time for Medicare Open Enrollment. Then on October 13th, the Medical Director of UNC Healthcare (the university system where my partner and I went for medical care) sent their patients who are insured by that Medicare Advantage plan this letter:

We are writing to tell you about a possible change in your ability to use UNC Healthcare's provider network... UNC continues to work toward a new agreement with {this Medicare Advantage insurer}. However, {this insurer} is not negotiating in good faith.*

So much for "quality, value and service."

Up to the day I received that letter, I reveled in the freedom Medicare provides. I can work for myself as a writer and never have to worry about losing coverage or having a big increase in my insurance premiums. The healthcare professionals I consult had been in network and happy to accept my insurance. I am such a fan that I'd been saying for years that everybody—not just those over 65—should have Medicare. But suddenly, with that Friday the Thirteenth letter, it was time to learn how the sausage is made.

First off, in case you are turning 65 and about to choose a Medicare pathway, there are two basic ways to go, and it's a big fork in the road.

- One way is what I have: A Medicare Advantage plan through a private insurance company that contracts with Medicare.
- The other way is to choose original Medicare, and if you wish, layer on a Medigap plan through a private insurer for extra coverage.

The essential thing to know about this choice is that in most states, Medigap insurers are legally required take you as a client at a set premium when you turn 65, but can turn you down or charge a much higher premium if you change to this path later on. So the fact that I chose a Medicare Advantage plan when I was 65 limits my choices now.

Research has shown that most people who choose Medicare Advantage over original Medicare do not understand the implications of that choice. A study by KFF (formerly known as the Kaiser Family Foundation) found that the marketing practices of Medicare Advantage plans include implying that the ads themselves were government sponsored, and that original Medicare is somehow deficient. The advertisement blitz at Open Enrollment time is "marketing madness," according to the head of KFF. The Commonwealth Fund found that 19 percent of Medicare eligible persons received fraudulent phone calls or saw fraudulent advertisements for Medicare Advantage plans. And besides defrauding potential insureds, Medicare Advantage insurers have been accused of massive fraudulent claims against the government for payment of services not rendered.

As I found out the hard way, Medicare Advantage plans are free to add or drop in-network providers. Going out of network can involve substantially lower payments or denial of claims. And while Medicare Advantage plans can offer lower premiums than a Medigap plan layered on original Medicare, some hospitals are dropping Medicare Advantage insurers because their payments are slow or low.

So what to do next? I do not live in one of the four states (Connecticut, Maine, Massachusetts and New York) that provide legal protections to people wanting to switch from Medicare Advantage to a Medigap plan on top of original Medicare. I was therefore at another fork in the road.

- I could switch to a different Medicare Advantage plan, if there was one that continued to work effectively with my university healthcare system. And how long would that relationship continue? Who knows?

- Or I could switch to original Medicare, which would assure me of coverage for whatever doctor I choose. This was appealing—but because Medicare *per se* has no out-of-pocket cap, I could potentially incur high costs in later years if my medical care became complex. And at this point, how much would I pay for a Medigap supplement? I was long past the lower premiums guaranteed to a new Medicare enrollee.

In his letter to patients, the Medical Director of UNC Healthcare urged us to call the Medicare Advantage insurer and tell them to negotiate in good faith. How persuasive would this be, for a company so intent on maximizing profits that they've run afoul of the US government? But I did contact the insurer. I also wrote to AARP suggesting they rethink their link with this insurer, for whatever that was worth.

But my main focus was comparing the dollar costs of replacement plans. And for that purpose, an insurance agent specializing in Medicare plans turned out to be very helpful. He even suggested a plan that facilitated transferring to a traditional Medicare plan plus a Medigap plan with that new company at a reasonable rate after the first year.

Many Medicare Advantage plans offer perks like gym memberships to attract relatively healthy Medicare recipients whose medical expenses are low. But later, when patients need more expensive care, Medicare Advantage plans often deny services that traditional Medicare would have covered—even though the coverage is supposed to be the same. A *Wall Street Journal* investigation found that Medicare patients with more serious illnesses were much more likely to leave Medicare Advantage for traditional Medicare, generating a savings to Medicare Advantage plans estimated at six billion dollars from 2018 to 2022. That savings to the private plans meant that taxpayers were covering the expenses of the sickest patients, while Medicare Advantage plans profited from insureds with less expensive healthcare needs.

Medicare is great, but the private insurers that are entwined with Medicare are problematic. The next time I advocate Medicare for All, I will add, "That's *Original* Medicare for All."

CHAPTER 34
THE NEW IMPROVED PINK TAX

Much has been written about the Pink Tax, which, despite the name, is not an actual tax. It refers to the practice of charging more for products intended for sale to women, where a nearly identical product for men costs less. The same manufacturer may charge more for a pink razor than a blue one. A women's blouse will often be more expensive than a similar men's shirt. A salon may charge more for a woman to have her hair cut than a man. These gender-based surcharges have a real impact. A 2015 study in New York City found an average markup of 7% for women's goods and services. And the Pink Tax starts early. Studies have shown that toys marketed for girls cost more than similar toys marketed for boys.

The Pink Tax has been recognized since at least the 1990s. In response, several jurisdictions have pushed back on gender surcharges for goods, services, or both. The first bill prohibiting gender discrimination in the pricing of services passed in California in 1996. In 1998 a New York City Council bill prohibited gender-based price discrimination in hair salons, dry cleaners, and other businesses. However, attempts to control gender discrimination in pricing at the national level have not succeeded. Jackie Spier, who sponsored the 1996 California bill, introduced similar legislation without success when she became a US Congresswoman. In fact, attempts to repeal the only actual pink *tax*, a higher tariff on imported goods for women, also failed.

Once aware of gender-based price discrimination, we can limit its impact on our lives. We can buy blue toys for our granddaughters and find a salon with gender neutral pricing. But that 7% markup in the New York study is peanuts compared with the "Anti-Aging Tax" we encounter as older women.

In 2012, FDA issued a Warning Letter to L'Oréal, the largest cosmetics company in the world, ordering the company to stop using drug-like claims on cosmetics sold in the United States. At the time, L'Oréal advertised that "anti-aging" products costing as much as $132 were clinically proven to "boost gene's activity and increase the production of youth hormones." While FDA does not require approvals for new cosmetic products, claims to affect genetic activity require products to be approved as drugs.

But these L'Oréal creams could never have earned FDA approval because the claims were unfounded. In 2014, L'Oréal reached a settlement with the Federal Trade Commission under which the company agreed to stop deceptive advertising, including claims that their products could "crack the code to younger looking skin."

Yet the company continued to push the envelope. In 2021 a class action lawsuit alleged that L'Oréal sold a range of "anti-aging" creams with inflated prices. Company advertising claimed the collagen molecules in these creams "restore the skin's cushion" and slow the formation of wrinkles. But according to the lawsuit, these creams stay on the surface of the skin and do not affect wrinkle formation. The suit points out that the worldwide market for "anti-aging" products containing collagen was expected to reach $6.63 billion by 2025.

L'Oréal is far from alone in its attempts to exploit women's fear of aging. Indeed, there has been a bumper crop of lawsuits and FTC enforcement actions against manufacturers of a variety of "anti-aging" products. As of 2017, there had been at least 31 class action lawsuits and at least ten FTC enforcement actions in the previous five years.

The Anti-Aging Tax is the Pink Tax on steroids. "Anti-aging" is a marketing claim that enables companies to mark up prices and increase profits on moisturizers. These baseless claims appeal to magical thinking. An "anti-aging" cream cannot restore our youth any more than pink slippers will make us Disney princesses.

Pushing back on this marketing scam requires that we confront our own ageism in the same way pushing back on the Pink Tax requires that we confront our sexism. Why pay more for a pink razor when a blue one does the job? Why pay more for the same moisturizer just because the label says "anti-aging?"

After experiencing the wage gap all our lives, we now face more retirement years with lower Social Security and less savings than men our age. The last thing we need is to spend extra money based on marketing puffery. Next time you go shopping, buy yourself a blue razor and a tub of ordinary moisturizer. Your wallet will thank you, and so will your self-esteem.

CHAPTER 35
MONEY PROFILE
ELIZABETH WHITE

> *As a Black woman, I've navigated racism, sexism, and now ageism. These experiences have fortified my resilience, particularly as I observe friends encountering ageism for the first time.*
>
> —Elizabeth White

In the early 2000s, Elizabeth White enjoyed a comfortable upper middle class lifestyle. As a Harvard Business School graduate, she had worked with the World Bank and consulted with major commercial clients on women's employment rights. Having grown up in Germany, Italy, and Libya, she also supported big box stores to source products from Africa.

The 2008 recession decimated her career. An occasional consulting gig kept her not quite afloat. NextAvenue published an essay she wrote about her employment struggles as a well-qualified post-midlife woman. The essay resonated with other women and went viral. Elizabeth built on that article in her 2020 book, *55, Underemployed, and Faking Normal*. Along with personal stories, the book presents strategies and down-to-earth tactics for thriving in challenging financial circumstances. She also presented a TED talk which has been viewed by millions. Ideas like forming a Resilience Circle with others facing these challenges, exploring transferable skills, and looking at lower paying jobs as a way to make ends meet, helped many women and men face later life financial challenges.

These days Elizabeth is in her seventies and very involved with housing solutions for olders. She is a fan of intergenerational housing and of shared living spaces. She founded NuuAge CoLiving, an organization dedicated to lowering costs, combating isolation and building community.

Follow Elizabeth White on LinkedIn and Instagram. She also writes a column for PBS News Online, where she shares ideas for recovering from financial hardship.

PART EIGHT
PURPOSE

What is our purpose in older life, as individuals and in community? How is that purpose the same as for women in times past, and how is it different?

What are our obligations to ourselves, to our families, and to the greater society?

These chapters ponder the big questions for today and our future.

CHAPTER 36
THE GRANDMOTHER HYPOTHESIS

A Woman-Centered Theory

In the 1980s, American anthropologist Kristen Hawkes observed Hadza hunter-gatherers in Tanzania and realized that the older women spent their time collecting food for the village children. This freed up the mothers to have more children. Hawkes showed that in early human societies, assistance from grandmothers increased the odds of grandchild survival, which created evolutionary pressure for grandmothers to live longer. Hawkes hypothesized that the fittest grandmothers had the most grandchildren, which led to longevity well past menopause in humans (as opposed to other apes whose lifespan ends just after their childbearing years). As humans developed more complex cultures such as tools for hunting and gathering, grandmothers continued to ensure that children were fully taken care of and learned the value of cooperation. After all, it is cooperation that defines the value of grandmothers in evolution.

Perhaps not surprisingly for such a woman-centered theory, there was opposition to Hawkes' work. This led Hawkes and others to formulate a mathematical model that demonstrates the presence of grandmothers doubles the human lifespan in under 60,000 years. Other researchers have expanded on the Grandmother Hypothesis, showing that physical and mental robustness later in life are uniquely human and tied to the value of older women.

Moving Our Bodies after Sixty

A more recent concept, the Active Grandparent Hypothesis, found that humans live longer if they move frequently—another difference from other primates. Other primates do not walk nearly as far as humans each day, and yet apes are unaffected by illnesses that plague sedentary people, such as cardiac disease. This suggests that humans were selected not just for longer lifespans but also for remaining physically active during that longer life, enabling us to care for the young. Staying active gives us the gift of time.

As women in the twenty-first century, how can we benefit from knowing that physical activity drives healthy longevity? To maximize our value to ourselves and the people we love, we must thrive and not just survive. And to that end, movement is essential.

Many of us find a joy in movement later in life that we did not know we had. Some of us (including me) hated gym class in school. Forced physical activity turned us off. After sixty we can discover (or rediscover) the joys of swimming, dancing, and lifting weights. That joy is for its own sake, not to impress others or make us look like models. We can relish movement and the ways it benefits our health regardless of body size and abilities.

These days, some of us have grandchildren while others do not. Even for those of us with grandchildren, our contact may be limited by distance. We can become sources of wisdom for one another and for our collective grandchildren, those coming up after us. We should, and do, have the freedom to define our own value and our own roles in retirement. And that freedom comes with a condition: That we continue to move our bodies.

Gloria Steinem famously said that women are the only people who become more radical with age. Our self-acceptance is radical in a society that marginalizes older women. Our writing is radical in a society that fails to tell our vivid stories. We are hard to fool because we have lived long enough to witness every human failing. Our freedom is rare in a society that prizes overwork, and we can use that freedom to benefit our communities by volunteering, being active in churches and civic organizations. Taking care of ourselves enables us to make the most of this precious phase.

Revering Older Women

As we define the meaning of our lives past menopause, we see that whether or not each of us is biologically a grandmother, we are here to pass on what we have learned through our decades of life.

We live long after menopause because grandmothers in past ages were essential to humans becoming complex, long-lived, social beings. These years when we may be liberated from our earlier roles as caretakers and workers gives us the power to make positive changes in our own lives, in the lives of our families, and in the larger culture.

CHAPTER 37
INCLUDING OURSELVES IN THE CIRCLE OF CARE

Three of my children were preschoolers at the same time. If you've lived through that phase of life, you probably don't remember much because you were too busy coping to store away memories. I do recall women whose children were already grown telling me to take care of myself; that I would be a better mother if I reserved time for me. I didn't have time to tell them I didn't have time. I didn't even have time to get annoyed.

All the same, I knew they were right. Back in college I had read *In a Different Voice*, Carol Gilligan's book about how women tend to care for everyone around us, excluding ourselves. Knowing that something is an issue may be the first step in making change happen but it doesn't mean you have time to act.

My children are long since grown. When their urgent needs subsided, I learned to take better care of myself in fits and starts. But something else has taken on the urgency of my children's needs when they were little: the cares of the whole world, which seems to come apart before our eyes. Other women's children are shot by random gunmen while entire species are dying. It is a different kind of constant pull: instead of a cry from the next room, a continual barrage of terrible stories on social media, in the newspaper, on television. Like a mother of young children who cannot rest while any of her children needs something, each of us is subject to the needs of our planet and the beings who live and die here.

There is nothing in this or any other book that will feed one child, stop one bullet, or save one member of an endangered species. And given the state of the world, the inevitable question is whether my projects are worthy; whether encouraging women to be creative, to access our whole selves and claim our agency, has a legitimate place. Am I encouraging us to fiddle, an orchestra of Neros, while Rome burns? How can we justify self-care in this moment?

In her book, *How to Do Nothing: Resisting the Attention Economy*, Jenny Odell suggests we recalibrate our attention. She says the loud addictive voices of social media absorb us, as if our phones were car windows tempting us to rubberneck an everlasting accident, the world colliding with itself. The way to deal with it, Odell suggests, is not to delete our Facebook accounts and loudly proclaim it online. The answer is to change our relationship with information, to use it instead of being used by it. The answer is to pay attention to what works for us, as humans and as citizens of the world. Like the women who advised me to take care of myself while my children were young, Odell advises her readers to take care of ourselves so that we can respond more effectively to the needs of the Earth.

The world is not a crying baby in the next room. It is more immediate than that: it is the declining quality of the air in our lungs, it is pollution in our blood. Taking care of the planet *is* taking care of ourselves.

But each of us is also our own finite self, our own complex water balloon riding this big rock through time and space. Taking the time to write, or whatever we do to bring ourselves joy, recharges us for the struggles ahead.

Not everyone has the bandwidth to do this. For many women—grandmothers at the border, older women who work full time and barely get by, women with complex health issues and inadequate resources—daily survival takes all they have. But for those of us who do have time to make a difference, finding our joy does not rob us of the energy for the work ahead. Instead it sustains us so that we can do our part for the world, whether our next step is tutoring a child, registering a voter, or calling an elected representative.

To care only for our own well-being would be indulgent, but we can take better care of those around us if we first take care of ourselves. Let's go to the gym, take our vitamins, floss our teeth, and remember to play. Let's make ourselves strong to do the work the world requires.

CHAPTER 38
OK BIG OIL

One of my favorite cartoons shows a medieval king in a gold crown standing on castle ramparts with a robed advisor by his side. Down below, a crowd of angry peasants gathers to storm the castle, half of them armed with pitchforks and the other half with torches.

You don't need to fight them, the advisor whispers in the king's ear. *You just need to convince the pitchfork people that the torch people want their pitchforks.*

This brilliant cartoon explains everything from feudalism to populism. How did the Confederacy recruit poor whites to die for rich plantation owners? Divide and conquer. How do today's politicians cut taxes on the rich with the blessing of the poor? Divide and conquer. And believe it or not, this stratagem also explains a lot about ageism. How is that, you ask? Let me begin with a confession.

I've spent way too much time arguing with young people on social media who are convinced that each and every person over fifty is individually responsible for the ruination of the planet. The suggestion that these young men and women should respect their olders is of course a lost cause; I don't bother. Instead, I ask them to consider whether they themselves have ever driven a car or drunk water from a plastic bottle. But the young people I communicate with remain unconvinced by talk of a double standard. When I raise the idea that all of us are enmeshed in a systemic problem, I am drowned out by a chorus of "OK Boomer," a refrain I hoped would have died out long ago.

A study published by two Harvard University researchers documents that the push to frame climate change and planetary ruination as a matter of individual responsibility results from a massive advertising campaign launched and paid for by—you guessed it—Big Oil. The study documents a years-long, coordinated campaign to blame consumers for buying and using polluting products while at the same time industry found ways to drive up demand.

This sleight of hand was not invented by Big Oil. For decades, tobacco companies blamed smokers for lung cancer while simultaneously reformulating cigarettes to make them more addictive. Nevertheless it's a brilliant marketing idea: Climate change is not the fault of the people who make plastic bottles and gas guzzling cars. No, that's just capitalism: Companies can't help making the products that people want to buy. And no matter how long Big Oil has covered up evidence of climate change (Hint: forty years), the resulting planetary damage is the fault of the people who buy the products.

And guess who has been buying those planet-killing products the longest? The people who have been around the longest: the Boomers. So climate change is not industry's fault. It's the fault of those horrible nasty old people who once drove you to your Little League games. Who among us over age fifty can claim to have left no carbon footprint? How can we push back at industry when we are seemingly complicit? How to fight such an airtight argument?

This advertising campaign may be the height of hypocrisy, but it's a fantastic shell game. Somebody in marketing whispered in the ear of the CEO: *You don't have to leave the oil in the ground. You just have to tell the young that their parents are ruining the planet.*

So I have a new way to argue with the young who have drunk the KoolAid: Follow the money. Don't be a dupe of Big Oil. We are all in this together. Let's go after the companies that have lied to us, ignored evidence of climate change, driven up demand, and who now tell us they support the Paris Climate Accord while at the same time they drill more oil wells.

All this may sound persuasive, but I still have trouble getting the message across. I need a great big advertising budget. Or at the very least a clever cartoon.

CHAPTER 39
THE POWER OF LATE BLOOMERS

The attempt to disempower an American woman unfolds across her lifetime. She is sexualized as a young girl, loses her reproductive freedom as a young woman, takes on the "Second Shift" as a mother, and becomes invisible after menopause. Rendering women over fifty invisible is even more insidious because in reality age liberates us. Not only do we live longer than men, our healthspan is longer as well. Our energy is freed as our children establish independent lives. And when our original careers wind down, we can devote ourselves to projects of our choosing. This period of life is a rich asset for each of us and for society.

But the time of our natural power is stigmatized. In the workplace and in the culture at large, women are judged more harshly for the appearance of aging. We are deemed sexless and irrelevant in ways that men of equivalent ages are not. And if we dye our hair or take other steps to counter the visible signs of aging, we are judged for that as well.

None of this is inevitable. We know that in some cultures older women are revered. We know from anthropology that older women's roles in early human societies were essential to the development of human culture. And we see examples of powerful older women who begin new careers after their children have grown.

What does it take to be a visible and powerful older woman? It starts with each of us. We can claim our power, own our sexuality, and both radically define and accept our appearance. We can counter ageist self-talk with positive messages. We can each build a public persona that serves us. We can give ourselves permission to claim our passions and creativity. What else can we do to become powerful Late Bloomers?

- **Late Bloomers can take new initiatives in our own lives.** The interests and passions we set aside to take on careers and raise children are still there, waiting for us. So are new avenues to explore. Giving ourselves permission to grow and change after midlife is the single biggest challenge to invisibility.

- **Late Bloomers can honor and build our collective power as Crones.** We claim our agency not only individually but also through participating in organizations such as these:
    - The Grandmother Collective
    - The Writers' Lab
    - The Centre for Aging Better
    - Old School

Each of us can learn about efforts already underway and look for new initiatives.

- **Late Bloomers can work for the empowerment of women across the lifespan.** The disempowerment of women is a lifelong problem that requires lifelong solutions and cooperation across all ages. Older women have the perspective to see the importance of agency across the full lives of women. We can:
    - Support programs that empower children to set boundaries and say no.
    - Support efforts to ensure reproductive justice for women.
    - Support policies including parental leave and subsidized childcare that enable mothers to lead full lives.
    - Support efforts to ensure economic justice for older women.

- **Late Bloomers can celebrate the shift already underway in American culture.**
    - Our sheer numbers, our buying power, and our power to affect social policy are unlike anything in the history of older women. We are changemakers. Women like Joan Price (*Naked at Our Age*), Julia Louise-Dreyfus (Wiser than Me), and Geena Davis (The Geena Davis Institute) make change happen every day. There are highly placed older women in the sciences, in philanthropy, in education, shifting the direction of society.

We know that representation matters. When Geena Davis acted the part of the president on television, acceptance of the idea of a woman president rose among the general public. So who stands to lose by keeping older women invisible? And who stands to gain as we claim our agency? Let's keep asking these questions.

We have the perspective to see women's disempowerment as a lifelong challenge. The woman who cannot obtain reproductive healthcare today will age into the gray-haired woman who is overlooked. We can counter the several ways that society disempowers girls and women, including fighting for reproductive freedom. We are connected to one another in ways that were invisible in our youth. We must make those connections more visible—including through the culture of older women.

CHAPTER 40
PURPOSE PROFILE
MAGGIE KUHN

> *Old people and women constitute America's biggest untapped and undervalued human energy source.*
>
> —Maggie Kuhn

Maggie Kuhn loved her job as editor of *Social Progress*, a journal of the Presbyterian Church, but mandatory retirement laws forced her to leave on her 65th birthday in 1970. A lifelong activist, Kuhn organized a group of friends who had also been forced to retire. Together they created a new movement to combat ageism, racism, and militarism. As founder of the Gray Panthers, Kuhn was a charismatic figure who advocated for nursing home reform, ending forced retirement, and improving health care access.

The Gray Panthers' motto was "Age and Youth in Action," and the organization fought ageism across the lifespan. Kuhn opposed retirement communities as "glorified playpens." She rented out rooms in her Philadelphia home to young people for reduced rates in exchange for chores and companionship.

Kuhn took stances on many issues that affect older persons. She claimed that controversy about funding Social Security was a smokescreen designed to distract attention from bloated military spending and tax cuts for the rich. She criticized gerontologists for emphasizing the frailties of old age, and pointed out that research spending favored that negative view. At a White House meeting, she scolded President Gerald Ford for calling her "young lady." "I'm an old woman," she told him.

Kuhn published her autobiography, *No Stone Unturned*, four years before her death in 1995 at age 91. The book chronicles her active love life along with her activism, and provides vivid examples of her motto "Learning and sex until rigor mortis." Kuhn's memoir is an exuberant tale full of the life of the senses. She wrote, "For me, this is a glorious period of life. More than anything else, old age has fed my passions."

Given that most women live years longer than men, Kuhn proposed that older women should feel free to form sexual partnerships with younger men or with each other. Reflecting on a love affair with a much younger man, she wrote: "Our sexuality is so influential in determining who we are and how we relate to others. Indeed, it is the material of life and to deny it in old age is to deny life itself."

The Gray Panthers continue to be active, with 25 chapters across the United States.

∼

PART NINE
CULTURE

The culture of older women is growing by the day. There are novels with older women protagonists, podcasts run by older women influencers, and nonfiction books about everything from older women's sexuality to the biographies of women who came to prominence in later life.

To immerse yourself in these riches can subdue the Inner Ageist, leading to a longer and happier life. Read books, watch shows, and subscribe to online groups that celebrate the wisdom and power of older women. Pay attention to what resonates and explore the possibilities for your own next steps.

PART NINE
COURSE

CHAPTER 41
ONCE UPON OUR TIME

Think back on *Snow White* and her nameless wicked queen from 1937; *Cinderella* and her stepmother from 1950; *Sleeping Beauty* and Maleficent from 1959. What a terrible career path we girls were given: the progression from young/beautiful/passive/good, to old/ugly/strong/bad. Neither of these fixed combinations is something we would stand in line for as adults capable of critical thinking. But we were impressionable children when we first saw those films.

The messages in the Disney films were inescapable: Good boys are active but good girls are passive; the good are always beautiful; to age is a sin; and for a woman to embrace her power makes her evil. As little girls we were almost certain to aspire to goodness and passivity, and to reject aging and power. And these messages did not stop with the 1950s. Disney's *The Little Mermaid* (1989) features a good, passive, beautiful heroine up against perhaps the scariest Disney villain of all: Ursula, the hideous, white-haired, power-hungry sea queen, with creepy tentacles for legs. Given the prejudices of the modern age, this evil queen is also fat.

Looking back on my childhood in the 1950s and 60s, I am amazed that these movies were seen as good clean family fare, suitable for repeat viewing by little girls. Clearly our mothers were not analyzing the subtext or they would have dragged us, kicking and screaming, from the theater. But come to think of it, in the 1980s I let my own children watch Disney movies, and I didn't think twice about *The Little Mermaid*. The view is different now, as an aging Queen.

The nexus of ageism and sexism pits younger women against older women. It denies us the chance to work and grow together. Anthropologists have demonstrated that women live long because we have much to teach the young, but the cultural image of the evil older queen denies that. The passive, beautiful princess is separated from the wisdom and power of older women and redeemed by a man's kiss. While some Disney features included benevolent older females (such as the three feckless good fairies in *Cinderella*), there were no strong, good grandmothers in these films.

And then in 1995 along came a non-Disney heroine who shifted the Hollywood perspective. *Xena, Warrior Princess* featured a strong female protagonist who fought her own battles in mythological realms. Instead of being saved by a prince, she herself was mentor (and possibly lover) to her friend Gabrielle. Instead of conflating youth, beauty, passivity, and goodness, Xena was multidimensional. Her character could be arrogant and uncertain. She was complex and powerful in a way previously reserved for male characters. One San Francisco station advertised the show as "Xena: A Dominatrix the Whole Family Can Enjoy." Xena inspired a new generation of female action heroes, from Buffy the Vampire Slayer to Starbuck in Battlestar Galactica.

Xena's popularity may be one reason Disney Studios moved toward stronger young female characters in more recent animations. For example, Belle is an avid reader, even if she does have a touch of Stockholm Syndrome (*Beauty and the Beast*, 1991), Mulan is a Chinese woman warrior who saves her city (1998), and Moana is a diplomat, explorer, and future Polynesian chieftain with no plans to marry (2016). And breaking the *Snow White* "fairest of them all" mold, newer films feature princesses of color. But even these newer films exclude positive role models of aging.

The classic Disney villain tried to recapture her girlish beauty in later life, and this "inappropriate" claim to power was her downfall, every time. What we have yet to see is old/beautiful/strong/good: a Disney heroine who is sexy and powerful in her older years. This is our challenge: To create such stories, not only to benefit our granddaughters, but ourselves as well. Somewhere in me is a little girl who still believes that older women are evil in our power. As an older woman, I need to tell myself new stories, stories about women who are strong and good later in life.

Disney mined the Brothers Grimm fairy tales for enchanting stories that emphasize the power of male characters. But there are other sources to tap. In her novel, *The Bee and the Orange Tree*, Melissa Ashley describes the life of Marie Catherine d'Aulnoy, one of the *conteuses*: a group of French women during the reign of Louis XIV who invented the fairytale as a way to criticize the constrained lives of women in their time. D'Aulnoy's Prince Charming suffers lovesickness for Cinderella, her princesses court princes, her queens rule queendoms. These feminist fairytales were turned upside down by the Brothers Grimm, but we can reclaim them. We can look, too, to the old myths, such as the tale of Baubo[*] in Greek mythology: an older woman whose bawdy humor comforts the goddess Demeter on the loss of her daughter to the underworld. Demeter's laughter at

Baubo breaks the grip of winter and allows spring to return to the world.

Now imagine Xena, not as a Warrior Princess, but as a Warrior Queen who rules a city-state with strength and compassion in the company of her lover. Imagine Moana, not as a young chieftain but as an older wise chief who brings all her life experience to her role as leader (much like the character Naniska in *The Woman King*). Imagine yourself, not as a lovely young hippie princess but as an older beautiful storyteller with the bawdy wisdom of Baubo and the strength to tell your tale. Write your stories for the girl you once were and for the granddaughters of us all.

It is time to grow more tales of strong beautiful older queens for the sake of ourselves and our culture.

* Not coincidentally, my publishing imprint is Baubo Books.

CHAPTER 42
OLDFLUENCERS

The internet plays host to a fabulous crone ecosystem that includes bloggers, podcasters, fashionistas, publishers and dancers. Their verve and variety is inspiring. Here are just a few examples of the creators in our growing community.

Podcasts

With so many to choose from these days, there are podcasts for every aspect of life in our sixties. Look around the internet for choices, or start with some of these great options.

- **Wiser than Me** — Actress Julia Louis-Dreyfus' immensely popular show where she interviews such famous older women as Fran Lebowitz, Nancy Pelosi, and Jane Fonda. Louis-Dreyfus introduced her first episode thusly: "I'm going to talk to old ladies. I want to know how they do it, how they did it. How do they navigate aging and life? Give us some tips from the front lines."
- **Badass Women at Any Age** — Host Bonnie Marcus interviews women with inspiring stories to tell about their

personal and professional journeys. Bonnie is also an author and public speaker. Her book, *Not Done Yet*, is all about reclaiming confidence and building late-life careers.
- **The Call to Create** — Host Betsy Hills Bush celebrates the downfall of gatekeepers with this lively podcast about creativity in later life. She chats with late-blooming artists, writers, musicians and more.
- **Late Bloomer Living** with Yvonne Marchese is an upbeat show with conversations, tips and tricks for living our best lives.
- **Zestful Aging** with Nicole Christina — Nicole's guests include everyone from filmmakers to scientists, showcasing their talents in later life.
- **Boomer Banter** with Wendy Green explores the complexities of life, including topics like financial concerns, maintaining health, and navigating divorces and widowhood. It's the podcast that acknowledges both the challenges and opportunities of aging.
- **Age Blind** with Nancy Shenker is all about intergenerational collaboration. With more of us than ever living past the century mark, Nancy's guests are frank and sometimes risqué as they talk about the challenges we face and what olders and youngers have in common.
- **Older Women and Friends** with Jane Leder aims to dispel the myths and explore the many contributions made by our age cohort—with a dash of humor.
- **Sex Advice for Seniors** is hosted by Suzanne Noble, whose goal is to provide all we need to know to have a thriving, nourishing sex life as we age.

Substack

When I started my Substack, Creative Crones, in 2024, I had no idea how many brilliant older women writers and influencers I would find there. Substack is a community as well as a place to read great writing. Women comment on one another's columns, send each other notes, and support one another's work. Check out what's available on the site; here is a sampling.

- Rona Maynard, the popular author of *Starter Dog*, holds forth about writing, her fifty year marriage, and life in general in **Amazement Seeker**, her articulate Substack column.
- Sari Botton writes **Oldster Magazine**, where she explores what it means to travel through time in a human body. She publishes personal essays and interviews with fascinating people like Cheryl Strayed and 92-year-old author Hilma Wolitzer.
- **The Granny Who Stands on Her Head** is author Ann Richardson's column, where she writes about growing older, emotions, the body, culture, and dying. And, yes, at 82 Ann does indeed stand on her head.
- Susan Orlean, 69, is a staff writer for *The New Yorker* and has published numerous books, including *The Orchid Thief*, which was made into the Academy Award winning movie *Adaptation* ("Yes, I was played by Meryl Streep; yes, it was weird"). Susan's Substack, **Wordy Bird**, covers fashion, writing, and the world at large.
- Jody Day, who founded the childless movement, writes **Gateway Elderwomen**, a Substack column about aging in a female body, rooting out internal ageism, confronting the 'Who's going to take care of me when I'm old?' issue, and developing intergenerational relationships.
- Every Sunday, Avivah Wittenberg-Cox publishes **Elderberries**, where she muses on what it's like renewing and deepening work, family and purpose in the 3rd Quarter - the years from 50 to 75.

LinkedIn

If you think LinkedIn is only for ambitious youngers, think again. LI is a hotbed of anti-ageism activism and a great place to network with others past sixty. The women on LinkedIn are savvy, tuned in, and incredibly mutually supportive. Here are just a few of the many worth following.

- **Janine Vanderberg** is an anti-ageism activist with Changing the Narrative.
- **Brooke Warner** is a TEDx speaker and the publisher at SheWrites Press, a leading hybrid publishing house that primarily features older women authors.
- **Jacynth Bassett** is an anti-ageism activist with Ageism is Never in Style.
- **Eleanor Mills** is founder of Noon, an organization in Great Britain that advocates for women past midlife. Her book is *Much More to Come*.
- **Mariann Aaldi** is an actress and TEDx speaker who reflects on the intersection of ageism, sexism and racism.
- **Helen Hirsch Spence** is a later-in-life entrepreneur dedicated to changing the narrative about ageing and developing longevity literacy skills.
- **Ashton Applewhite** is an activist extraordinaire, founder of Old School, and the author of *This Chair Rocks: A Manifesto Against Ageism*.

Online Magazines

There are online magazines for women over sixty covering every subject, from travel to work to money. Here are a few of my favorites.

- *Certain Age Magazine*
- *CrunchyTales Magazine*
- *Persimmon Tree*
- *NextAvenue*

- *Kuel Life*

Each of us can find our favorite topics and our community of women in this developing culture. The influence of women over sixty is steadily growing, and so are our connections in community. We become stronger as we weave those connections together. Enjoy!

CHAPTER 43
THE VIBRANT PEN

Older women writers are putting us front and center in stories and novels. Nonfiction books include everything from photography (such as *Wise Women: A Celebration of their Insights, Courage and Beauty*) to studies of mythology (such as *Goddesses in Older Women*). And there is a rich vein of fiction and memoir to choose from. Plus with the advent of indie publishing, the gatekeepers are scrambling to keep up with the demand for books and stories about women after sixty. It's a grand time to be a writer—or a reader!

Novels

Ruth O. Saxton is professor emeritus of Mills College in California, where she founded the Women's Studies program in the 1970s. In 2020, when Saxton was eighty, she published *The Book of Old Ladies*, her analysis of how older women are portrayed in fiction. Saxton talks about the "Little Red Riding Hood" phenomenon in fiction from back in the day: The older woman is in the story, but her story doesn't matter (she is "fodder for the wolf"). But in recent years more women are writing vivid, complex older female characters.

Here are some of Saxton's recommendations for books with strong older women protagonists.

- Sarah Ladipo Manyika was born in Nigeria and lived in many countries before settling in San Francisco. Sarah's slender novel *Like a Mule Bringing Ice Cream to the Sun* tells the story of Dr. Morayo da Silva, a retired English professor approaching her 75th birthday. Each of the novel's twenty-one chapters is a first-person account by Morayo or someone she encounters in her neighborhood. We observe her love of color, beautiful African fabrics, and bright red lipstick, as well as her kindness, her curiosity, her love of books, and her delight in driving her Porsche, Buttercup, on San Francisco's hills.
- Isabel Allende's *The Japanese Lover* tells of another San Francisco denizen, Alma Belasco, whose parents sent her from Poland in 1939 to live in safety with relatives in an opulent San Francisco mansion where she met Ichimei Fukuda, the son of the family's gardener. The reader gradually learns about a secret passion that has existed for nearly seventy years. *The Times* describes this lovely book as "a novel of high romance and lush sensuality, unashamedly about the enduring power of love and ending on a note of grace."

Saxton also recommends Octavia Butler's *Kindred*, Paula Marshall's *Praisesong for the Widow,* and my own *Brilliant Charming Bastard,* the tale of three women scientists in their sixties who take smart revenge on a lying dilettante who is dating all of them and stealing their ideas. Saxton calls *Bastard* "an upbeat read with a happy ending."

Non-Fiction

Nonfiction books about older women push back on sexism and ageism with facts and well-reasoned argument. Here are some of my favorites.

- *This Chair Rocks: A Manifesto Against Ageism* by Ashton Applewhite. This groundbreaking book is full of essential information about ageism and how to combat it, both within ourselves and in society at large. No wonder Ashton's TED talk has been viewed by millions.
- *Breaking the Age Code* by Dr. Becca Levy. Levy is a lead researcher at the Yale University School of Public Health. Her team has investigated the effects of ageism for years. She shares her findings in this informative book, including that older persons with a positive view of aging live an average of 7.5 years longer and in better health.
- *55, Underemployed, and Faking Normal* by Elizabeth White. Let go from her prestigious position at the World Bank in her mid-fifties, White shared the too-common experience of hiring discrimination. She parlayed her financial expertise to craft a new way of living fully with limited means, which she shares in this savvy book.

Nonfiction can also enhance our spiritual and philosophical approach to life in our sixties. Here are some books that can expand our perspective.

- *Women Rowing North* by Mary Pipher. Drawing on her experience as daughter, sister, mother, grandmother, clinical psychologist, and cultural anthropologist, Pipher explores ways women can cultivate resilient responses to the challenges we face. "If we can keep our wits about us, think clearly, and manage our emotions skillfully," Pipher

writes, "we will experience a joyous time of our lives. If we have good maps and guides, the journey can be transcendent."
- *The Queen of My Self* by Donna Henes. In this reinvention of archetypes, Henes points out that the frequently quoted trio of Maiden/Mother/Crone lumps together all women past midlife. She proposes a new model of Maiden/Mother/Queen/Crone to recognize the powerful life stage from midlife to cronehood.
- *Goddesses in Older Women* by Jean Shinoda Bolen. Bolen followed her bestselling book, *Goddesses in Everywoman*, with this volume focused on the pantheon of older goddesses and their traits, including compassion, outrage, laughter and wisdom.

Creative Nonfiction

Exploring later lives well lived opens us to possibilities. Here are some stellar examples to explore.

- Billie Best has been a music producer, a marketing executive, a farmer and a writer. Her memoir, *How I Made a Huge Mess of My Life (or Couples Therapy with a Dead Man)*, is a witty, unblinking look at success, failure, bliss, life, and death. Best's story of caring for her dying husband while coming to terms with his infidelity is enlightening and engaging.
- When Rae Padilla Francoeur wrote *Free Fall: A Late-in-Life Love Affair*, she did not know of other older women writing about sex. Yet her memoir features bedroom scenes of unparalleled power. She immerses us in the visceral experience of a late life love affair, and then explores the countervailing pull of the narrator's responsibilities to her career and to a demanding family life. If you have been ambushed by lust after sixty (or want to be), if your desire

has gone off like fireworks in the lives of the people around you, this story is sure to resonate.

These are just a few of the marvelous books for and about us. As you find your own favorites, please drop me a line at stella@stellafosse.com. Building our connections in this great new culture is essential.

CHAPTER 44
SEE IT THEN BE IT

Geena Davis did not worry about all those stories of movie roles drying up for women in their forties until it was her turn. After making a movie every year throughout her career and starring in huge box office hits like *Thelma and Louise* and *A League of Their Own*, the actress made one movie in the entire decade of her forties. Just one. And, she says, it was not because she was fussy.

Then after her daughter was born, Davis realized how few female characters there were in children's programming. Davis started talking with friends about sexism in children's shows, but few had noticed. The shortage of females onscreen (including older females) was an invisible problem. Davis was determined to make it visible. She sponsored the largest study ever undertaken on depictions of gender in children's television and G rated films. The results of the study showed there were three male speaking roles for every female role, and only 17% of people in crowd scenes were female. According to Davis, the ratios had not changed since 1946. One reason may be that studio decision makers are still overwhelmingly white men.

And yet, unlike the representation of women in Congress, the representation of women on screen could be changed instantly. Davis believes that if we represent women in the media in realistic numbers, acting in powerful and interesting ways, it will change how society views women and change our role in the culture. She has evidence for this claim from her own career: One study showed that people who watched Davis star as President of the United States in the 2005 show *Commander in Chief* were 67% more likely to vote for a female presidential candidate than before they watched the show.

Davis decided to use her financial resources and her status in the industry to push for change. In 2004, she founded the Geena Davis Institute, which conducts research and advocates for greater representation of women and racial minorities in television and movies. Because of her prominence, Davis has access to people all over the entertainment industry and has conversations about unconscious bias whenever she can.

Regarding the nexus of ageism and sexism, Davis brings data to the table. *Frail, Feeble and Forgotten: A Report on the Movie Roles of Women of Age*, a study of 2019 films, showed that women over 50 were underrepresented. And when they did appear, women over fifty were frequently depicted as frail or homebound. Older women were four times as likely to be shown as senile compared with older men. Only one in four films studied passed the Ageless Test, which requires that films feature at least one female character over 50 who is essential to the plot and portrayed without reducing them to ageist stereotypes.

An expanded study, *Women Over Fifty: The Right to Be Seen Onscreen*, analyzed movies from 2010 to 2020. This study found older characters were more likely to be shown as villains, less likely to be included in romantic storylines, and that while older characters in general were underrepresented, older females were much less prevalent than older males.

Women, especially older women, also face bias when they work in the film industry as actors, directors, producers, and in technical roles. Davis' 2019 film, *This Changes Everything*, is a full length documentary told in the words of women in media about their experiences with bias.

Like Geena Davis, actress Meryl Streep has the connections and resources to champion older women in Hollywood. In 2016 Streep decided to use her influence to support women screenwriters over forty through her project, The Writers Lab. Since that time, Oprah Winfrey and Nicole Kidman have added their clout to the project. The Lab is a four-day development workshop that gives women screenwriters the opportunity to work intensively on their scripts with the support of established writers, directors, and producers. Through one-on-one meetings, panel discussions, guest speakers, and group meals, mentors and writers engage in a rigorous process that provides support in the craft and commerce of screenwriting.

Geena Davis believes, with justification, that what we see onscreen is powerful. When we present women in power positions onscreen, suddenly the question becomes, *Why not in real life*? Her slogan is, "If she can see it, she can be it."

Movies and Shows

Geena Davis' work on behalf of representation in Hollywood is bearing fruit. Here are just a few of the growing number of movies and shows that reject stereotypes in favor of portraying the vivid lives of women after midlife.

- *The Woman King* stars Viola Davis as General Naniska, leader of the Agojie, a historical all-women warrior band who protected the kingdom of Dahomey from slavery in the 17th to 19th centuries. Davis brings incredible intensity to her role. The ensemble of women warriors following a powerful crone into battle is groundbreaking, as is the subject matter of an African nation successfully defending its people from enslavement.
- *The Good Fight* is Christine Baranski's vehicle to bring political awareness to the character of Diane Lockhart, which she originated in the long running series *The Good Wife*. Baranski is sophisticated and assertive in her role as a powerful litigator.
- *Hacks* is a celebration of women comedians of a past age who did not receive the recognition they deserved. It stars Jean Smart as the seventy-year-old Deborah Vance, reinventing herself in tandem with a much younger woman comedian. The *New York Times* declared, "Jean Smart is having a third act for the ages."
- *Grace and Frankie* premiered in 2015 and ran for seven fabulous seasons. Jane Fonda and Lily Tomlin are brilliant as women whose husbands of forty years fall in love with each other, leaving their wives to build a new life together despite their very different styles. Along the way, Grace and Frankie start a company to sell a vibrator specifically designed for older women.
- *Good Luck to You, Leo Grande* is a stunning exploration of older women's sexuality. Emma Thompson stars as a woman past midlife who has never had an orgasm and hires a younger and very wise sex worker to engage in brave exploration.

There is much to explore in our culture of vibrant women past midlife: blogs, newsletters, podcasts and more. We have spent a lifetime absorbing gendered ageist messages, and to consult powerful women's voices helps us push back on those messages. Much like pulling weeds in a garden, we can root out negative messages and plant positive ones.

Each of us co-creates this culture. What are you called to do, to please yourself, enlighten your friends, and help shift the dominant narrative?

CHAPTER 45
CULTURE PROFILE
DR. RUTH SAXTON

I wanted to read the novels in which fictional older women prepare for the journey of aging, inhabit the territory, and become increasingly their truest selves.

— Ruth O. Saxton

Dr. Ruth O. Saxton is a Professor Emerita of English, co-founder of the Women's Studies program, and founder of the Rhetoric and Composition program at Mills College in Oakland, CA where she was recognized for over forty years of exemplary teaching.

Her scholarly books include *The Girl, Constructions of the Girl in Contemporary Fiction by Women; Approaches to Teaching Woolf's Mrs. Dalloway* (with Eileen Barrett); and *Woolf and Lessing: Breaking the Mold* (with Jean Tobin). Her most recent work, *The Book of Old Ladies: Celebrating Women of a Certain Age in Fiction* explores the aging female protagonist in contemporary fiction.

She was teaching and in the process of starting on the *Old Ladies* project when a car accident left her visibly unscathed, but with a traumatic brain injury. A neurologist who evaluated her for head trauma told Saxton that level of function was what she should expect at her age. Dr. Saxton's reflections are below.

> "When I lost my brain as I had known it in a car accident in my early sixties, I wanted stories of development and hope to counter the dismal medical advice to quit my job and accept that I might not ever read or write again. I am not given to denial, but I do have a streak of defiance when faced with dire predictions. Rather than give up, I spent years of hard work—physical therapy, speech therapy, occupational therapy, vision therapy, psychotherapy, acupuncture, Pilates—while impersonating my former self at home and at work. When my reading improved from its second-grade level, I returned to my original project knowing first-hand the importance of hope and reinvention after loss. I am committed not to regaining a lost "whole" self, but to embracing the possibilities and new modes of knowing that the self I am in makes possible."

With a great deal of support and hard work, Dr. Saxton learned new ways to be. *The Book of Old Ladies* was published during COVID lockdown in 2020. Saxton continues to lead workshops on older women's fiction in Oakland, California, where she enjoys life with her family and dog, and has started a creative writing class. She is figuring out new ways of navigating as she loses her sight, continuing to embrace new modes of knowing and being.

∽

PART TEN
SPIRIT

Our perspective can shift in our sixties as we become more aware of mortality. We may reassess priorities and decide to focus on what is dear to us: the people we love and the passions that matter most. We consider our legacy and how we wish to be remembered. And above all, we do not let mortality be the enemy of the now; gratitude for each new day is paramount.

CHAPTER 46
RETIREMENT TILL THE END

> *You can think of death bitterly or with resignation, as a tragic interruption of your life, and take every possible measure to postpone it. Or, more realistically, you can think of life as an interruption of an eternity of personal nonexistence, and seize it as a brief opportunity to observe and interact with the living, ever-surprising world around us.*
> —Barbara Ehrenreich in *Natural Causes*

Retirement is a lovely vacation that ends in death. Our exhilaration when we first retire is tempered by how it will end. Back when I was working, if I had two weeks off, I reveled in the first week and spent the second week dreading the return to the office. Even then I knew that was absurd. *Why not enjoy it all?* And I don't want to do that again: Dreading the end of this lovely retirement vacation rather than immersing myself in its everyday magic.

Yet permanence is scary. Each night of the week before I married, I dreamed I was making love with a different man. Beautiful men, imaginary men, in the most romantic settings: On the beach, in a hot air balloon, on a linen-clad table in a private dining room. Marriage terrified me. "Till death do us part" meant I was already with the last man I would ever make love to. Things did not turn out that way; the marriage produced wonderful children but did not endure.

After I quit my last full-time job, I kept dipping my toe in consulting, partly because money is nice and partly because I did not want to face the finality of retirement. But consulting lacks the appeal of a tryst with a handsome man. I am finished with consulting; I have grown intolerant of corporate bullshit.

So, then, mortality. Retirement till the end.

I've never been sanguine about death. I spent my sixties counting the years from my current age to the average age at death of my closest female relatives. I reassured myself that my remaining years were longer than the entire lifespan of a woman in the Middle Ages. But American lives are shorter now, thanks to the pandemic and its impact on healthcare. And my health is not what it was when I turned sixty. So, what is the zip code of the state of denial?

Making sense of death is complex. The idea that one's consciousness will vanish—poof—is hard to fathom, even if you have sat with the dying, even if you have undergone surgery where consciousness was suspended for hours. Yet I have no quarrel with the fact that I did not exist before I was born. Why should death seem any different?

There is a wonderful scene in *The Lion in Winter* when Katherine Hepburn as an aging Eleanor of Aquitaine and Peter O'Toole as an aging Henry II ponder the nature of life and death. They compare human life to a lost bird that flies out of darkness into the open window of a great hall, passes through light for a moment, then flies through the opposite window and back into darkness. The philosopher George Yancy put it this way: "I feel trapped between two infinities of meaninglessness."

My cousin in her nineties sent a wonderful holiday card back in 2021, replete with pictures of great-grandchildren. She thinks of faith as the comfort of earlier generations; her comfort is in these children, in the chain of life over the centuries. *This is what matters,* she wrote in her card. And that, I think, is the crux of it: to find what matters for each of us as we confront the mystery of time and the majesty of death.

Professor Yancy conducted a series of interviews with philosophers and theologians. Each of them had a different idea about what matters in the face of mortality, grounded in their respective traditions.

A Buddhist scholar said that self-obsession and the insistence on seeing ourselves as separate from the universe is the root of our fear. Instead, like my cousin, we can see ourselves as part of a continual process of regeneration. If we accept that change is constant, we can make the most of the present.

A Jewish scholar traced the complexities of responses to death in Jewish texts. Two of the ideas he described were the sense that the individual life is part of a long, collective story; and embracing mortality as a portal to more fully embrace our finite lives.

A Christian theologian believes that love continues, through everyone we have loved, long after we ourselves are forgotten. She also believes that she will be reunited with her loved ones after death, including her mother, who died of ALS. During the interview, Dr. Yancy challenged this idea by quoting Stephen Hawking who also died of ALS and who once said, "I regard the brain as a computer which will stop working when its components fail... There is no heaven or afterlife for broken down computers; that is a fairy story for people afraid of the dark." The Christian replied that even if we are not reunited, as love we live forever.

A scholar of Yoruba tradition explained that in that faith heritage, the spirit knows how long it will live on earth before he or she is born but loses that knowledge at birth. At death the spirit returns to that same otherworld, and the meaning of the person's death depends on whether they fulfilled their purpose in life.

A Muslim historian said in that tradition, fragments of the self exist for as long as God maintains Heaven and Hell. And good works are part of the decision God makes about the soul's destination.

An atheist philosopher resolves the paradox of finding meaning in a finite life by pursuing two parallel paths: On the one hand, making plans for projects that hold meaning, and on the other, living each day with the understanding that none of those plans may come to pass because today is the only day we can be sure of.

These interviews gave me a sense of being part of a broader community now and across time, struggling to find meaning. Feeling that connection helped me gain some serenity about mortality. Each interview added to my understanding of what it means to live each day in this life we are given. As a writer, I love the idea that fragments of the self persist. In her classic text, *Writing Down the Bones*, Natalie Goldberg said that when we write, we ride the universe as it moves through us. We write because how we lived is important. "Let it be known, the earth passed before us." And I embrace the idea that the meaning of our death depends on whether we fulfilled our purpose. As a partner and a mother, I love the idea that love persists even after we are gone, even after we are forgotten. As an egotist and a neurotic, I appreciate the importance of accepting change, accepting the loss of control, and making plans that may be futile.

Two of Jack Kerouac's precepts for writers were: *Accept loss. Be in love with your life.* I hear those together as: *Love this thing that we know will disappear. Love it fully, with a whole heart.* W.H. Auden enjoined us to dance till we drop. And what else can we do but dance, each to our own purpose, if we are to live each day of this last-in-a-lifetime, lovely vacation.

You've heard the saying, "Don't let the perfect be the enemy of the good." It is just as important not to let mortality be the enemy of the now. Instead let us make mortality the ally of the now. Let the mutual recognition of our collective destiny make our time together more precious.

CHAPTER 47
A LIFE IN REVIEW

> *Healing the past liberates the future to be a mystery rather than a rerun.*
>
> —Vicki Robin from "Coming of Aging" on Substack.

It's December and we are down to the essentials. Outside the branches are bare, while inside the house, the packages are shipped and the cupboards empty as we make ready for holiday travel. The New Year is almost upon us with chances for new resolutions, new activism, new growth. This liminal time is perfect for reflection. I am taking a class with a death doula, and one of the assignments is to review our lives, the ups and downs, for each era from birth until now.

The instructions claim that conducting a life review can increase our satisfaction with life. We can revisit our accomplishments, find closure with issues that feel unresolved, and arrive at new contentment. By revisiting our relationships we can deepen our understanding of their meaning.

A formal Life Review can happen in conversation or through writing. Therapists trained in life review may ask questions like, "When were you first attracted to another person?" or "What wisdom would you like to share with the next generation?" When memories are difficult, a facilitator can suggest a reframe to help deepen their meaning. Another method is to use writing as a tool to review our lives, either in a group or individually. That is what we are doing in the death doula class.

I did a similar exercise years ago, when a friend invited me to co-lead workshops based on *Telling the Stories of Life through Guided Autobiography Groups* by Birren and Cochrane. The book asks participants to record their turning points: the moments when a decision or an external event altered our trajectory. The process continues with writing on themes rather than chronologically. Another book that is organized by themes, *Writing Your Legacy* by Campbell and Svensson, is great for solo writers. Using photographs is yet another way to access our memories. So is listening to music we enjoyed at different eras in life. The group my friend and I led continued sharing and writing long after the scheduled workshops ended.

This time, for the death class, I wrote by decades about the big events of my childhood, my teens, and so on until my sixties. What stands out is how dense my life has been. So many startling and unexpected events. So many twists and turns in relationships with parents, ex-spouses, children, friends. Such a kaleidoscope. My life is not so much a narrative arc as a picaresque tale with one episode after another and a cast of recurring characters. I was always striving to find something, and in my sixties I found it. But what was it that I found? Peace? Fulfillment? The end of ambition? A truce with my Inner Critic? Distance from regrets? Or perhaps just a focus on what I'm going to do with each precious day.

Another way to find meaning is to write legacy letters to family members. A legacy letter is a personal statement about what we have learned in life and why we value our relationships with loved ones. Anyone, writer or not, can write a legacy letter, to preserve memories and express gratitude to those we love. Some people write one legacy letter, and some write individual letters to each child and to others who have been important in their lives. Legacy letters let folks know your hopes for them, and how you hope they will remember you. You can decide when to share these letters, or leave them with your important papers for distribution at the end of your life.

My ability to find meaning, to develop equanimity about who I am and what I have accomplished, is enhanced when I take the time to reflect. And after different versions of a life review made years apart, I see the value of revisiting the process at various stages in life. Each time I review my life, I give myself the gifts of peace and understanding. I recommend taking time for these reflections.

CHAPTER 48
SPEAKING BAWDY OF THE DEAD

I'm going to dance in all the galaxies.

—Elizabeth Kugler-Ross

My mother died in 2020 on Pandemic Thanksgiving, just shy of 95. She had spent the last two years of her life in hospice, in a nursing home. Most of the last year of her life, the virus cut her off from family and visitors. She did not die of COVID. She was blessed to have care staff who moved into the facility and locked themselves away from their own families to keep the residents safe. Such a gift cannot be measured. I like to think Mom would have done the same, had there been a pandemic in her earlier years, when she was Director of Nurses in a care facility.

Mom was a nursing student in Chicago during World War II. Because so many nurses were on the front lines, Mom and her classmates went to school in the daytime and worked nursing shifts at night. In the last year of her life, when she and I were on the phone most days, she told me about a young man she dated after nursing school. She loved it when he drove her around Lake Michigan with the top down on his convertible. When she broke up with him she told him she was only dating him for his car. Until that moment I had no idea that Mom had ever been a Mean Girl.

But there was certainly more to her than her staid nurse-and-mother image. One day in the 1960s when I was a teenage nerd on the couch with my nose in a book and Mom was ironing her nursing caps, she started laughing and put down the iron. I asked her what was going on.

"I just remembered a poem I hadn't thought about in years." She recited it from the ironing board.

Under the spreading chestnut tree
The village idiot sat,
Amusing himself by abusing himself
And catching it all in his hat.

Another time Mom insisted on telling a lurid tale from a book she was reading on the history of Hollywood. Some movie star from the 1940s was known for wearing metal dildos to parties. She had never heard of such a thing. I was a *Steely Dan* fan by then and didn't find it quite so startling.

After my dad left in the 1970s Mom led a quiet social life. I wonder what her life would have been like, had there been online dating sites when she was in her fifties and sixties. She did have one fling with a pharmacist, and it amused her no end that love came back into her life for a time after midlife.

In her last years when she lived in the nursing home, she liked to talk about a handsome doctor who visited her. And when I published *Aphrodite's Pen*, my book encouraging post-midlife women to write erotica, Mom was so amused that she insisted on keeping a signed copy by her bedside. By then her vision was poor and I don't think she read it, but she loved the idea.

There are stories of anyone's life that don't make the cut for the memorial service. We don't speak ill of the dead and we also don't speak bawdy of the dead. But the romantic lives of our forebears were as vivid and complex as our own and deserve their own memorial. The dead are real and their stories are real. It's part of our role as wise old women to be the storytellers and to keep the tales alive from generation to generation.

Mom would have agreed with Oscar Wilde that life is too important to be taken seriously, and perhaps death is too important as well. On the day Mom died, an old friend of hers had just walked up the driveway of the care home for a visit at Mom's window, calling her name and wishing her a Happy Thanksgiving. Mom took a deep breath, as if she had run a long race, and breathed her last. As the staff closed the window shades out of respect, Mom's friend stood in the driveway, shaken and not sure what to do. The owner of the care home drove up just then, dressed head to foot in a turkey costume. She said to Mom's friend, "I wish I could hug you and comfort you." But this was Pandemic Thanksgiving, no turkey hugs allowed.

STELLA FOSSE

My wish for all reading this is that when we are separated by illness or necessity we remain connected in every way we can, by phone and letter and video call. That we tell stories to broaden and deepen our connections, especially the bawdy stories, the funny stories, the moments that will make us smile in years ahead.

The poet Muriel Rukeyser said the universe is made of stories, not of atoms. And so is love, and so is memory.

CHAPTER 49
MY NEXT LIFE BUCKET LIST

> *I have a next life bucket list: More sex, better singing voice, the ability to tan.*
>
> --Billie Berlin, in *Aphrodite's Pen: The Power of Writing Erotica after Midlife*

I don't believe in reincarnation. I don't believe in much, except an objective external universe and that our task in life is to apprehend it. So I've been startled lately, when confronted with the ills that flesh is heir to, to find myself thinking: *That will be fixed when I get my next body.*

This strange idea may be why I love Billie Berlin's concept of the Next Life Bucket List. Billie wastes no time on regrets. She's not beating herself up for some rude thing she said twenty years ago, or wondering what would have happened if she'd changed college majors in 1970. Her list has just one focus: An attribute wish list for when she revisits this orb.

Billie has many fantastic qualities: great energy, a fine wit, and a terrific acting talent. When I imagine my own next life, much of what I'd like to be I've finally become. I know when to speak up and when to walk away. I have a fully functioning BS detector. I understand how to string words together on a page.

But why wait until I'm older? I'd like to speak my mind earlier in life, even as a kid. I'd like to possess the perspective I now enjoy, but starting in my teens. I'd like to start writing books in my twenties so I could fit more books into my allotted span. Many of us are Late Bloomers, enjoying our best lives after sixty, and that group definitely includes me. But if I could do anything, be anything, right from the start, my Next Life Bucket List might include things like this:

- **Good manners**: Definitely lacking in this lifetime. Is it easier to be gracious with a couple million in the bank? Are good manners a luxury enjoyed by the rich? So it has always seemed to me. Or is that just an excuse for my curmudgeonly ways? When I lived in New York in my twenties, I attended parties with the descendants of robber barons. I still recall their poise, their understated dress, and their ability to engage people of different backgrounds in meaningful conversation. Of course their old money was new money once, generations ago. Thinking back, I wonder if that smooth gentility was a distraction from a history of exploiting marginalized workers. Could I acquire just a smidge of that polish without the ruthless backstory? Something to aim for, next time around. Or do I have it backwards: Do good manners lead to wealth? A five year

study of the newly rich showed that certain behaviors we associate with good manners are actually networking skills that lead to financial opportunities. Habits like sending thank-you cards, remembering people's birthdays, and introducing one's self properly in social settings lead to better financial outcomes. Wait for my next life? Or should I cultivate manners now?
- **Optimism**: Happiness and emotional intelligence are traits of optimistic people. But is it possible to be smart and optimistic? Some research suggests that optimism is associated with lower cognition and poor decision making. That's because humans have an inborn tendency to absorb information that is favorable to them and ignore unfavorable information. It takes strong critical thinking to overcome that bias. But on the other hand, unrealistic pessimism about our older years based on internal ageism shortens lives, according to research by Dr. Becca Levy and others. Another reason to focus on objective reality. So never mind the unfettered optimism. On my next visit to Earth I'll keep my skepticism but order a pair of rose-colored glasses.
- **Fine motor coordination**: Women who can sit in a meeting and crochet without looking at their hands amaze me. Surely this is an unrecognized superpower.

Maybe who I already am is pretty much okay. Maybe I can spruce up my social skills without dying first. And unbridled optimism might be overrated. As Lily Tomlin said, "No matter how cynical you get, it's hard to keep up." But being able to crochet without looking down? I'll take that one in a heartbeat.

And so, to whatever part of my brain thinks I'll be issued a new body when this one goes kaput, get cracking on those fine motor skills. You have at most a few decades to line up the next life.

But perhaps I should say "please" to myself and practice my manners.

CHAPTER 50
SPIRIT PROFILE
ALUA ARTHUR

By envisioning who I want to be on my deathbed, I invited life in.

—Alua Arthur

Alua Arthur is the founder of Going with Grace, an organization that focuses on compassionate support for persons at the end of life. Alua was born in Ghana and had early experiences with death when her family fled a murderous coup d'etat in the 1980s. As an adult, she advocated for her dear brother-in-law while he was dying of lymphoma. This experience led Alua to her calling as a death doula, a role she had not heard of but could tell was needed. As a "recovering attorney," she brings to her clients a wide range of skills, assisting with business matters and medical directives, as well as the unfinished emotional business that can come up at the end of life.

The role of a person to shepherd others through the death process is ancient and revered. This concept has become more prevalent in

Western countries in the 21st century. Death doulas can provide both spiritual and practical guidance including helping to plan memorial services, assisting with advance directives, and providing emotional support to the terminally ill person and their family.

Alua's book, *Briefly Perfectly Human,* calls readers to get in touch with something deeper in life, even before we near its end. In her popular TED talk, "Why Thinking about Death Helps Us Lead a Better Life," Alua asks this question: "What must I do to be at peace with myself so that I may live presently and die gracefully?"

And of being with the dying, Alua says, "It's utterly profound. Getting to witness the doorway to existence is a gift and a privilege and a huge honor. Hopefully we can continue to treat it as such."

∼

EPILOGUE

What a wonderful life I've had. I only wish I'd realized it sooner.

— Colette

This book is a retrospective, looking back on essays I wrote in my sixties from my current vantage in the early days of the next decade. So now that I'm in my seventies, here is a totally unscientific preview of coming attractions, for the benefit of all you freshly minted sixty-year-olds.

When you've met one seventy-year-old, you've met one seventy-year-old. But after an informal survey of friends my age, we do share certain traits in common.

At sixty I felt pretty much immortal, while at seventy my body reminds me that I am mortal after all. Given the history of every human who has ever lived on this planet, my mortality should not have been news, but it was.

Perhaps because of those reminders, I am even clearer about how I want to spend my days. That doesn't mean I resent folding laundry, because I don't. It is more a matter of finding contemplation in the ordinary life of cooking breakfast and going for a walk.

I am glad to focus on the things I prize most, which means hanging out with people I love, supporting my favorite causes, and writing books. At the same time, I am less attached to outcomes. If I got too sick to create the rest of the books on my To Be Written list, I'd be glad for the ones I did write. I notice that shift in attitude with my peers as well, both writers and non-writers, as ambition wanes and gratitude grows.

I've read that in the Jewish tradition, there are two deaths: when a person stops breathing, and when their name is last spoken by someone who remembers them. I suppose for a writer there is a third death: when the last person reads the last copy of their last book. Even the advent of Print on Demand (so that books no longer go out of print) won't stop that third death forever. The key thing is to make peace with impermanence. I'm still working on that one; perhaps it's a goal for my eighties.

What can *you* expect in your seventies? Alas, my crystal ball is in the shop. But if your seventies turn out anything like mine, the forecast is for greater perspective and continued joy. I love Leonard Cohen's line, "Ring the bells that still can ring." At seventy there are plenty of bells to ring. May that be true for all of us, and may it continue.

QUESTIONS TO THINK, WRITE, AND TALK ABOUT

Consider these questions solo or with friends.

If you are in a reading group, you are cordially invited to contact Stella Fosse's publicist, Graham Bird, to schedule a time for Stella to meet your group online for conversation: graham@stellafosse.com

Part One: Power

- If you were to invent a strong older woman character for a story, what traits would she have? What would be her goals?
- Be mindful of ageist stereotypes in newspaper reporting and elsewhere. Consider writing a letter to the editor when you encounter an egregious example.
- The word "Crone" originally meant a withered old woman, but the word has been reclaimed to mean "Crown:" the crowning achievement of a woman's life to become a wise matriarch. What does "Crone" evoke for you?
- Watch Ashton Applewhite's "Let's End Ageism" TED talk. What comes up for you?

QUESTIONS TO THINK, WRITE, AND TALK ABOUT

Part Two: Creativity

Try these writing prompts:

- Write an Anti-Bucket List of everything you are no longer willing to do.
- When I am an old woman, I shall dye my hair purple.
- At fifty she had no lovers. At sixty she had three.
- She walked into that room like the ancestors sent her.
- "Women have a special corner of their hearts for sins they have never committed." —Cornelia Otis Skinner
- Try writing a limerick—here's an example:

    A dirty old woman from Rome
    Took all of her lovers straight home.
    Wasting time out to dinner
    Is just for beginners;
    You never know when they will roam.

(See *Aphrodite's Pen* for more limerick ideas and examples.)

Part Three: Sexuality

- Consider your thoughts and feelings about masturbation now and when you were younger. What has changed in your outlook, and what remains the same?
- Think about a sexy scene in a book you have read or a movie that you have watched. Write a story about it with yourself as the protagonist.
- Read one of Joan Price's books or online columns on older sexuality and highlight ideas that appeal to you.
- Watch *Good Luck to You, Leo Grande*, and write about your reactions. Or organize a watch party with friends and talk about the movie afterwards.

QUESTIONS TO THINK, WRITE, AND TALK ABOUT

Part Four: Healthcare

- Prepare for your next doctor visit by drafting a Medical Summary Sheet (See Chapter 16).
- What are your views on menopausal Hormone Therapy? How did you arrive at those views?
- In your experience, which medical interventions have been most (and least) helpful?
- Discuss your preferences about healthcare with the person you might designate as your decision maker, if and when you are unable to advocate for yourself.

Part Five: Body

- Consider the ways your body has served you well.
- What positive memories do you have about your face and its features over the years? What do you like about it, when you look in the mirror now?
- Try Walking Meditation. Walk slowly through a beautiful place, noticing each step and what is around you.
- Dance to music in your living room, either standing or seated.
- Taste a favorite food with your eyes closed. Savor each bite.

Part Six: Beauty

- How important is personal style to you? How has that changed (or not) over time?
- Do you enjoy dressing playfully? How do you like to show off?
- At this point in life, do you use color to play with visibility, whether it's with tinted conditioner, tinted moisturizing cream, bright clothes or jewelry? What else would you like to try?

QUESTIONS TO THINK, WRITE, AND TALK ABOUT

Part Seven: Money

- Watch Elizabeth White's TED Talk. What comes up for you?
- What kinds of part time employment would appeal to you?
- How would you spend your days if money were no constraint?
- Is downsizing in your future? What plans are you considering?
- How does a shared housing scenario sound to you?
- What does your retirement budget look like? Have you consulted a financial advisor?

Part Eight: Purpose

- Take a look at online pages for organizations that support human rights for older persons. Which are you drawn to join or support?
- What form of self-care would you like to add to your day?
- Review the Profile of Maggie Kuhn at the end of Part Eight. Which issues that she fought for remain relevant today?
- If you were to choose one policy issue to focus your energies, what would it be, and why?

Part Nine: Culture

- Choose an example of older women's written culture (such as a book or blog) to read and reflect upon in writing.
- Watch a movie about an older woman and notice the ways her age was affirmed or denigrated by other characters.
- Share some of your favorite examples of older women's culture with your friends, or recommend a selection to your book club.
- How would you like to enrich the culture of older women,

QUESTIONS TO THINK, WRITE, AND TALK ABOUT

through your own creativity and through supporting other creators?

Part Ten: Spirit

- When did you first become aware of death? How did that awareness affect you at the time?
- What have been some major turning points in your life?
- What have you always wanted to do that you have not yet done? How can that knowledge inform life going forward?
- Watch Alua Arthur's TED Talk "Why thinking about death helps you live a better life." What comes up for you?

FOR FURTHER READING

Part One: Power

- *This Chair Rocks: A Manifesto Against Ageism* by Ashton Applewhite
- *Breaking the Age Code* by Dr. Becca Levy
- *Age Ain't Nothing but a Number: Black Women Explore Midlife*, edited by Carleen Brice
- *Ageism Unmasked* by Tracey Gendron
- *In Our Prime: How Older Women are Reinventing the Road Ahead* by Susan J. Douglas

Part Two: Creativity

- *It's Never Too Late to Begin Again: Discovering Creativity and Meaning at Midlife and Beyond* by Julia Cameron
- *The Vintage Years: Finding Your Inner Artist After Sixty* by Francine Toder
- *Bird by Bird: Some Instructions on Writing and Life* by Anne Lamott
- *Write & Sell a Well-Seasoned Romance* by Stella Fosse
- *Aphrodite's Pen: The Power of Writing Erotica after Midlife* by Stella Fosse

Part Three: Sexuality

- *Naked at Our Age: Talking Out Loud about Senior Sex* by Joan Price
- *Sex For One: The Joy of Self-Loving* by Betty Dodson
- *Mating in Captivity* by Esther Perel
- *Fifty First Dates after Fifty* by Carolyn Lee Arnold
- *Polyamorous Elders: Aging in Open Relationships* by Kathy Labriola
- *The Dirty Old Women Anthology* edited by Lynx Canon
- *Writing Ourselves Whole* by Jen Cross

Part Four: Healthcare

- *Natural Causes: An Epidemic of Wellness, the Certainty of Dying, and Killing Ourselves to Live Longer* by Barbara Ehrenreich
- *Elderhood* by Louise Aronson, MD
- *Estrogen Matters: Why Taking Hormones in Menopause Can Improve Women's Well-Being and Lengthen Their Lives—Without Raising the Risk of Breast Cancer* by Avrum Bluming, MD, and Carol Tavris, PhD

FOR FURTHER READING

- *Unwell Women: Misdiagnosis and Myth in a Man-Made World* by Elinor Cleghorn

Part Five: Body

- *Killers of a Certain Age* by Deanna Raybourn
- *The Diet-Free Revolution* by Dr. Alexis Conason
- *The Obesity Paradox* by Dr. Carl Lavie
- *The Body is Not an Apology* by Sonya Renee Taylor
- *Unapologetic Aging: How to Mend and Nourish Your Relationship with Your Body* by Deb Benfield (December 2025)

Part Six: Beauty

- *How to Be Old: Lessons in Living Boldly from the Accidental Icon* by Lyn Slater
- *Iris Apfel, Accidental Icon: Musings of a Geriatric Starlet* by Iris Apfel
- *Stepping Out: The Unapologetic Style of African Americans Over Fifty* by Connie Briscoe
- *Advanced Style* by Ari Seth Cohen
- *Wise Women: A Celebration of Their Insights, Courage and Beauty* by Joyce Tenneson
- *Visible: 60 Women at 60* by Jenny O'Connor

Part Seven: Money

- *55, Underemployed, and Faking Normal* by Elizabeth White
- *Rebellious Aging: A Self-Help Guide for the Old Hippie at Heart* by Margaret Nash
- *With a Little Help from Our Friends: Creating Community as We Grow Older* by Beth Baker
- *The Senior Cohousing Handbook* by Charles Durrett and Patch Adams

Part Eight: Purpose

- *The Fountain of Age* by Betty Friedan
- *Older, Wiser, Fiercer: The Wisdom Collection* by Carol Orsborn, Ph.D.
- *Not Dead Yet: Feminism, Passion, and Women's Liberation* edited by Renate Klein and Susan Hawthorne
- *Social Policy for an Aging Society* by Carole B. Cox
- *No Stone Unturned: The Life and Times of Maggie Kuhn* by Maggie Kuhn

Part Nine: Culture

FOR FURTHER READING

- *The Book of Old Ladies: Celebrating Women of a Certain Age in Fiction* by Dr. Ruth Saxton
- *Kindred* by Octavia Butler
- *Free Fall: A Late-in-Life Love Affair* by Rae Padilla Francoeur
- *Write & Sell a Well-Seasoned Romance* by Stella Fosse
- *Women Over Fifty: The Right to be Seen Onscreen* by the Geena Davis Institute
- *Like a Mule Bringing Ice Cream to the Sun* by Sarah Ladipo Manyika
- *The Japanese Lover Isabel Allende*

Part Ten: Spirit

- *Women Rowing North* by Mary Pipher
- *Briefly Perfectly Human* by Alua Arthur
- *Goddesses in Older Women* by Jean Shinoda Bolen
- *The Queen of My Self* by Donna Henes
- *Hagitude: Reimagining the Second Half of Life* by Sharon Blackie

ACKNOWLEDGMENTS

This book was written without my knowledge.

—Zadie Smith

In November 2023 I attended a workshop led by Patrice Gopo called "Greater than the Sum of the Parts: Transforming Personal Essays Into a Book." Based on her experience publishing two essay collections, Patrice shared the hows and wherefores of turning disparate essays into a coherent whole. The "herding cats" metaphor featured prominently.

I had quite the collection of cats. I had been blogging for years about life in our sixties as well as writing essays for other publications. I had also drafted half the chapters for a book about life in our sixties (co-author Steeviejane Parks was writing the other chapters). When our vision for that book diverged, we shut down the project and my chapters became available for a different use.

As Patrice made clear, crafting a book from heterogeneous materials takes far more than slapping a cover on a hodgepodge of stuff. The process involves identifying throughlines, balancing variety with continuity, and keeping the book coherent and interesting whether readers skip around or read straight through. Then there are gaps to be filled by writing new material. If I've in any way achieved those goals, it's been with the help of these wonderful folks:

- Patrice Gopo, many thanks for sharing your expertise and your methods
- Graham Bird, thank you for being my first reader, my publisher and my partner in life and art
- Diana Rosinus, thank you for always creating the best book covers
- Steeviejane Parks, thank you for suggestions about the chapters I wrote for our erstwhile project
- Ashton Applewhite, your Old School Office Hours meetings never fail to provide new ideas and perspectives on this vivid older life
- Jaki Shelton Green and Ruth Saxton thank you for your passionate and insightful interviews, excerpted in your Profiles.

When a first take of this manuscript was complete, a team of early readers gave invaluable advice that spanned the full range from content to typos. Teri Brown, Betsy Bush, Padget Gerler, and Karen Smiley, I cannot thank you enough for your insights. The remaining faults in this book are my own.

I also want to thank the podcasters and interviewers who have spoken with me over the years and expanded my thinking about the meaning of life in our sixties. The Crones I've interacted with on Substack, on social media, and through your comments on my blogs have each added to my understanding. Also, thanks to the other venues that previously published versions of some of these essays.

It takes a village to write any book, and in the case of this book, it's taken a whole city—and a whole decade. Thanks and hugs to you all.

ABOUT THE AUTHOR

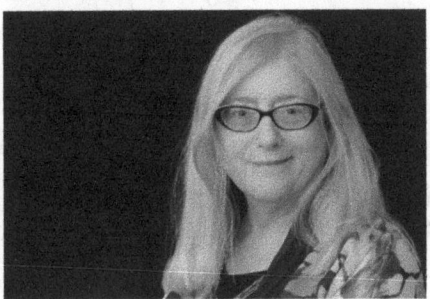

Stella Fosse

Stella Fosse is the *nom de plume* of an author whose backgrounds in finance and biotechnology have informed her essays for the past decade. Stella began writing sexy stories in her sixties as a creative antidote to the ageism and sexism older women face in society. She champions older women's creativity by leading workshops, and invites other women authors of a certain age as guest bloggers on her website.

Stella is a frequent guest on podcasts for women past midlife. She has been published in many online venues. Stella also blogs about issues of interest including creativity, romance, and older women's health on her website and on Substack.

Her most recent book, *Write & Sell a Well-Seasoned Romance*, empowers women to tell vivid stories of late life love. Traditionally published works include her book *Aphrodite's Pen: The Power of*

Writing Erotica after Midlife. Stella's linked stories, *The Erotic Pandemic Collection*, is an imaginative exploration of romance in quarantine. Her first novel, *Brilliant Charming Bastard*, is a nerdy, romantic escapade through the San Francisco biotech scene. Her second novel, *Vampires of a Certain Age*, expands her exploration of the vivid lives of older women.

Stella's books are available at your local bookseller and your favorite online place. She shares her writing, as well as ideas and resources for empowering women past midlife, at www.stellafosse.com.

Please join Stella on social media here:
    BlueSky: https://bsky.app/profile/stellafosse.bsky.social
    Facebook: https://www.facebook.com/StellaFosseAuthor/
    Instagram: https://www.instagram.com/stella.fosse/
    LinkedIn: https://www.linkedin.com/in/stellafosse/
    Substack: https://stellafosse.substack.com

www.ingramcontent.com/pod-product-compliance
Lightning Source LLC
Chambersburg PA
CBHW011408070526
44586CB00021B/2577